Diphtheria Serum as a Technological Object

Postphenomenology and the Philosophy of Technology

Technological advances affect everything from our understandings of ethics, politics, and communication, to gender, science, and selfhood. Philosophical reflection on technology helps draw out and analyze the nature of these changes, and helps us understand both the broad patterns and the concrete details of technological effects. This book series provides a publication outlet for the field of the philosophy of technology in general, and the school of thought called 'postphenomenology' in particular. Philosophy of technology applies insights from the history of philosophy to current issues in technology, and reflects on how technological developments change our understanding of philosophical issues. In response, postphenomenology analyzes human relationships with technologies, while integrating philosophical commitments of the American pragmatist tradition of thought.

Titles in the Series

Diphtheria Serum as a Technological Object: A Philosophical Analysis of Serotherapy in France 1894–1900, by Jonathan Simon

Digital Media: Human-Technology Connection, by Stacey O. Irwin

Acoustic Technics, by Don Ihde

A Postphenomenological Inquiry of Cell Phones: Genealogies, Meanings, and Becoming, by Galit P. Wellner

Postphenomenology and Technoscience: The Manhattan Papers, edited by Jan Kyrre Berg O. Friis and Robert P. Crease

Postphenomenological Investigations: Essays on Human–Technology Relations, edited by Peter-Paul Verbeek and Robert Rosenberger

Design, Meditation, and the Posthuman, edited by Dennis M. Weiss, Amy D. Propen, and Colbey Emmerson Reid

Diphtheria Serum as a Technological Object

A Philosophical Analysis of Serotherapy in France 1894–1900

Jonathan Simon

LEXINGTON BOOKS
Lanham • Boulder • New York • London

Published by Lexington Books
An imprint of The Rowman & Littlefield Publishing Group, Inc.
4501 Forbes Boulevard, Suite 200, Lanham, Maryland 20706
www.rowman.com

Unit A, Whitacre Mews, 26–34 Stannary Street, London SE11 4AB

British Library Cataloguing in Publication Information Available

Library of Congress Cataloging-in-Publication Data

Names: Simon, Jonathan, 1964- author.
Title: Diptheria serum as a technological object : a philosophical analysis of serotherapy in France 1894–1900 / Jonathan Simon.
Description: Lanham : Lexington Books, 2016. | Series: Postphenomenology and the philosophy of technology | Includes bibliographical references and index.
Identifiers: LCCN 2016046931 (print) | LCCN 2016050329 (ebook) | ISBN 9781498531474 (cloth : alk. paper) | ISBN 9781498531481 (Electronic)
Subjects: LCSH: Diphtheria—France—History—19th century. | Diphtheria—France—History—20th century. | Serotherapy—France—History—19th century. | Serotherapy—France—History—20th century.
Classification: LCC RM138.6.F8 .S56 2016 (print) | LCC RM138.6.F8 (ebook) | DDC 614.5/123—dc23
LC record available at https://lccn.loc.gov/2016046931

♾™ The paper used in this publication meets the minimum requirements of American National Standard for Information Sciences—Permanence of Paper for Printed Library Materials, ANSI/NISO Z39.48-1992.

Printed in the United States of America

Contents

Acknowledgments

With special thanks to Volker Hess, Axel Hüntelmann and Ulrike Klöppel for the DFG project on serotherapy. Thanks also to Viviane Quirke, Christian Bonah, Bernadette Bensaude-Vincent, Jean-Paul Gaudillière and Andrew Feenberg for their input on an earlier version of this book. To all the librarians and archivists who helped along the way, in particular those at the Pasteur Institute in Paris and at Garches. To my colleagues in Lyon; Nicolas Lechopier, Jérôme Goffette, Evelyne Lasserre, Hugues Chabot and Olivier Perru. To Patricia and Owen for their support and patience. To Lilly and Pollux for not breaking the computer.

Archives Consulted

I would like to acknowledge the use of material from the following archives:

Archives de l'Assistance Publique - Hôpitaux de Paris, Archives de l'Académie des Sciences, Archives de l'Institut Pasteur, Archives Municipales de Lyon, Archives Municipales de Paris, Archives Municipales de Nancy, Archives Municipales de Grenoble, Archives Municipales de Bordeaux, Archives Municipales de Montpellier, Archives Municipales de Marseille, Archives Départementales du Rhône-Alpes, Archives Départementales de Lorraine, Archives Départementales du Val de Marne.

I consulted the following newspapers and reviews for the period concerned:

Le Figaro, Le Matin, La Semaine médicale, Lyon médical, Bulletin médical, Bulletins et mémoires de la Société médicale des hôpitaux de Paris.

Chapter 1

Medicine as Technology

What would it mean to take a medical drug seriously as a technological object? In this book I aim, if not to answer, at least to address this question using a particular historical example—serotherapy for the treatment of diphtheria in France. The reader will quickly understand that the approach developed here is largely historical, entering into considerable detail concerning the production, distribution and use of serum at the end of the nineteenth century. Nevertheless, the guiding question remains philosophical, and turns around the concept of a technological object. While, as we will see in what follows, the notion of a technological object is poorly defined, we aim to show how thinking about a medical drug in terms of technology rather than integrating it into a typical narrative of drug innovation as a scientific endeavor can open up new analytical perspectives. In trying to place the drug as technology, we will start with the process of its manufacture from raw materials and finish with a reflection on its political significance in late nineteenth-century France. We will, therefore, be considering not so much the drug's physiological interaction with the human body, but more the sense that it took on in the professional, social and political context into which it was introduced.

Serotherapy, an innovative treatment for diphtheria dating from the end of the nineteenth century, was initially developed in Germany. Nevertheless, it was rapidly introduced across Europe, in the Americas and in Australia, with local production providing for national demand in most of these countries. In this book, I will be focusing on the anti-diphtheria serum in France, and will discuss the production in neighboring countries only insofar as it affected the French case. Thus, rather than providing a typical historical study of the development and introduction of a new therapy, I want to understand what was important in the specific configuration of the production and use of the serum in France, exploring the local particularities in greater detail than a classic narrative of scientific innovation would permit. Indeed, one important argument I will be making is that the full sense taken on by the serum for patients, their families and medical professionals, as well as for the wider population differed from country to country. French serum was not, in the end, the same as German, Italian or American serum.

From the outset I am positioning myself with relation to an old debate in the philosophy of science. 'Classic' philosophies of science promoted the universality of science, with a scientific method or fact being universally either true or false.[1] Carried over into the domain of pharmaceutical innovation, medical drugs are considered to be effective or ineffective against a disease, independently of the context in which they are administered. This universalist conception of the medical drug is foundational for the elaborate modern system for testing and approving such products, with the randomized clinical trial its trademark practice. Indeed, one of the last critiques a contemporary pharmaceutical researcher would think of launching against a clinical trial would be the geographical location of the plant where the drug was manufactured or the country where the manufacturer had its head office.[2]

This argument concerning the specific nature of French serum fits into a wider approach in the philosophy of technology. Thus, based on this study of the serum we intend to launch a reflection on what it means to think about a medical drug as a technology in general. While certain aspects of serotherapy are very specific to this case and do not translate to other medical drugs, even other sera, a number of considerations can be generalized to the majority of drugs sold and consumed today. Thinking of such medical drugs as technological objects can serve not only to make them more visible as objects in healthcare today but also allow researchers in the social sciences to question the various functions of such drugs in modern society. This is a valuable exercise in itself, given the ubiquity of prescription and over-the-counter drugs in our lives today. The analysis of the medical drug as technology opens up areas that are not immediately obvious subjects for the history of these products, with the second half of the book launching into wider considerations of the role of national and regional identity as well as state power in the definition and perception of these objects. In the end, our reflection on the medical drug as a technology leads us deep into historical territory often considered beyond the scope of philosophy of technology.

MEDICINES, MEDICINE, AND TECHNOLOGY

Medical technology has interested historians of medicine for a number of decades. As an area of study traditionally dominated by doctors, history of medicine was to a large extent constructed around narratives of the great medical practitioners and revolutionary medical innovations which contributed to the constitution of the modern medical sciences. A mounting interest in patient-centered histories and other versions of social history of medicine in the second half of the twentieth century turned attention away from this kind of hagiography and toward the day-to-day practice of medicine in the past. With the development of such studies focused on the second half of the nineteenth and the beginning of the twentieth century, historians struggled to assess the clinical significance of certain key medical technologies around the turn of the century, particularly in the hospital setting. Thus, for example, the discovery of X-rays and their almost immediate adoption in the domain of medical imagery led to a transformation in diagnostic techniques starting at the turn of the century, in a period where much older technologies, such as the stethoscope and the thermometer were also establishing a central place in medical practice.[3] It is not hard to find histories of the medical technologies that were either invented in this period, like X-rays, anesthesia and antiseptic devices, or that developed out of earlier innovations, like the stethoscope. These histories, reflecting the tradition of the history of medicine written by doctors, are usually hagiographic, and have often been written by specialists in the medical field subsequently forged around the object in question.[4] Nevertheless, professional historians of science have also looked at these medical technologies from different perspectives, trying to evaluate the ways in which they transformed the practice and perception of medicine, particularly hospital medicine, at the turn of the century. Joel Howell's in-depth analysis of technology in a Philadelphia hospital has become a classic in this field, with other studies filling in different features of this landscape.[5] There have also been several studies of ensembles of technologies, such as Thomas Schlich's treatment of organ transplantation and a collected volume edited by Carsten Timmermann and Julie Anderson on medical technologies more generally.[6]

While it is not original, then, to consider the place of technology in the history of medicine, particularly in this key period of the second half of the nineteenth century, this is, to my knowledge, the first book to treat a medical drug as a technological object rather than as a transparent means to deliver a treatment, whether effective or not.

This is not to say that technology is absent from the history of pharmacy. When one thinks of the development of pharmacy across the twentieth century, the images that come to mind are of production rooms filled with large steel fermentors (often adapted from models developed for the brewing industry) producing antibiotics or vaccines and of conveyor belts bearing thousands of identical pills to be dropped into bottles, the whole process free from the contaminating presence of human operators. Other machines stick on labels and package the bottles in boxes ready to be dispatched for sale and use. This image of pharmaceutical production, proudly brought to the fore in the industry's promotional literature and films after World War II, contrasts with the vision of the apothecary's laboratory from the eighteenth century where the artisan-apothecary is hunched over a mortar or crucible manually preparing his own wares. Indeed, the twentieth century has witnessed an inversion of the image of quality in pharmacy. The personal care associated with manual artisanal production of medical drugs (including the harvesting of the raw materials) that traditionally served as a guarantee of the quality of the products bought at the pharmacy has since been replaced by new conceptions and standards of quality associated with a sterile human-free mass-manufacturing environment and the production of raw materials by chemical synthesis or purification. In this sense, the high-tech production environment is central to the representation of the difference between 'modern' and 'traditional' pharmacy.

A particularly striking example of this technological image typical of modern pharmacy, is the production of penicillin dating from World War II, where American industrial manufacturers like Merck developed dedicated deep fermentation technology in order to be able to produce penicillin in the quantities demanded by the American war effort. Looking at archival photographs of Merck's facilities we can see quite clearly how a pharmaceutical production plant from 1945 resembled other industrial installations in post-war America.[7] While it was during this period that the pharmaceutical plant came to resemble other industrial manufacturing sites, the logic of mass production that was behind these kinds of factories had been introduced much earlier. Indeed, serum production, as we shall see in detail in this book was a form of industrial manufacture of a medical drug that already broke with the artisanal traditions of the apothecary, and the serum was far from being the first mass-produced drug in Europe or the United States.[8]

It is not difficult to argue for the crucial role played by technology in the development of penicillin as a medical drug, with the introduction of antibiotics as we know them today depending on important technological developments. The breakthrough in terms of production capacity came with the passage from surface to deep fermentation.[9] Thus, the first experimental production of penicillin by Norman Heatley in Howard Florey's laboratory at Oxford relied on surface fermentation of the *Penicillium* mold using a modified bedpan. Confined to the surface of the liquid in the vessel, the quantities of the mold and hence its product were limited. Although innovative and ingenious, Heatley's method did not succeed in producing sufficient penicillin to save the life of reserve constable Albert Alexander, the first experimental subject to be treated with penicillin at the Radcliffe infirmary in Oxford in 1941. Penicillin became a significant medical drug only following the engagement of American industry to produce it industrially under pressure from the wartime administration.

Although, as we have already remarked, serum for the treatment of diphtheria was produced on a large scale using what might be described as industrial methods, it is not my aim here to put a great deal of emphasis on this aspect of the history. Once again, I want to analyze the drug itself as a technology, placing the technology that surrounded its production to one side except insofar as it was constitutive of the drug. This reflection applies equally to the pharmaceutical form of the serum. Historians have only recently started studying this important question of the different forms of medical drugs and how they changed over time, notably with the rise of the industrial manufacture of these products.[10] The serum that I will be considering in this book was produced and distributed in liquid (and later desiccated) form for administration by intraperitoneal injection, but I will not be excessively concerned with this dosage form or with the means of delivery either, as for me these are secondary technological issues that risk distracting from the central focus which, once again, is thinking about the medical drug itself as a technology. This being said, it would have suited my purpose just as well, if not better, if this material therapy had assumed a more familiar modern pharmaceutical form as either a pill or a capsule. As Jeremy Greene has rightly pointed out, the pill—as a pharmaceutical form—is particularly rich in its signification.

> The pharmaceutical tablet is the perfect image of health care as commodity: a compact unit of therapy, portable, exchangeable across borders, universalized in shape to a nearly spherical form, its therapeutic value having nothing to do with the local circumstances of administration (unlike a surgical procedure or an injection) and having everything to do with a highly abstract network of data, research, and therapeutic information of which it is both product and emissary.[11]

Indeed, it is quite surprising if we consider the ubiquity of the pill or tablet in modern life, that it has not been the focus of more studies in the history or philosophy of technology. Like the standardized container used in the international transport of goods the pill or tablet has been both an element in and a force behind the standardization of drug delivery that has changed the relationship we have with health and disease.[12] Be that as it may, my point here is that while technology is a subject that increasingly interests historians of medicine, and within this field, historians of pharmaceuticals as well, there has yet to be a sustained examination of the medical drug itself as technology. I presume that this failure to take the medical drug seriously as technology is largely to do with our intuitions about what counts as technology or more specifically what counts as a technological object.

Asked to draw up a list of technological objects we encounter in our daily lives, we would probably start today with computers and smartphones before moving on to vehicles (motorized and non-motorized). The list goes on. But the technological association is to do with the machine-like nature of the object itself, as well as the evident teleological dimension, and the deeper implicit sense of being a human product. That the medical drug is not obviously a machine, however, does not, in my opinion, disqualify it from having the status of a technological object. The obvious question to ask, then, is What is a technological object?

This is a question that philosophers of technology have regularly asked. Although we do not find any consensual definition of what counts either as technology or as a technological object in the philosophy of technology literature, most philosophers would agree that human intention and intervention are essential characteristics, but this minimal requirement leaves an enormous range of objects in the running. Recently, Joseph Pitt proposed an extraordinarily wide definition of technology as 'humanity at work,' which would clearly cover any manufactured drug, as well as a great many other objects and processes that we might not intuitively consider technological.[13] Although more detailed, Carl Mitcham's earlier definition of technological objects scarcely narrows down the field.

> Technology as object is the most immediate, not to say the simplest, mode in which technology is found manifest, and it can include all humanly fabricated material artifacts whose function depends on a specific materiality as such.[14]

On one hand, there is no doubt that medical drugs (modern or otherwise) conform to this definition of a technological object. But, on the other hand, unless one excludes living beings, considering them to lie outside the scope of this definition, it seems that nearly all the objects in our modern environment could be taken to be technological. To summarize, the problem is we have an intuitive idea of what constitutes a technological object but the rare definitions offered by philosophers are so wide that they encompass what most people would consider to be such objects and a whole lot more besides. It is, therefore, not very surprising that while a medical drug like the serum fits such an abstract definition of a technological object, it nevertheless lies at the margins of the group of objects generally taken to illustrate this term. Furthermore, histories of medical drugs like serum or antibiotics tend to be recounted on the model of histories of science rather than the model of histories of technology, with the focus of a large number of these works being on the science that went into the discovery of the 'active principle' and the story ends there. It is rare to find any discussion of the way a drug was produced on an industrial scale, let alone any protracted examination of the history of how the molecule, once discovered, was delivered to the organism through the powder, pill or liquid sold to doctors or the public.[15] What have traditionally interested historians of pharmacy are the pathways to discovering new molecules (particularly the ones that are considered significant innovations) and the elucidation of their mode of action. More common in recent work on the history of drugs, however, is a consideration of the social context into which these products were introduced and the effects that their dissemination, use, and abuse have had on society.[16] This is certainly a theme that I will be taking up in the story about serum in France, but oriented not so much to understanding the effects of new drugs on society as understanding how a particular social configuration informed the medical drug itself.

THE PHILOSOPHY OF TECHNOLOGY

Part of the problem of finding a useful, consensual definition of a technological object is that the philosophy of technology is a relatively young area of philosophical enquiry, and like many other rising subdisciplines in the humanities lacks a well-established canon. If we compare this field to the philosophy of science, for instance, the difference is striking. Whether one agrees with their positions or not, there is a lineage of authors (Compte, Whewell, Carnap, Popper, Kuhn to take just a limited chronological selection) that most members of the philosophy of science community would take as having made significant contributions to the development of the field.[17] While the majority of philosophers of technology today refer to Husserl, Heidegger, Marcuse, and Marx as pioneers and role models, they do not pretend that there is a group of thinkers who could serve as the founders of the field.[18] Indeed, no one from this list is primarily identified either as a philosopher of technology, or, for that matter, as a philosopher of science. Another observation we can make about philosophy of technology is that it is less well established institutionally than philosophy of science, with relatively few philosophy departments around the world promoting their programs in philosophy of technology.[19] These two observations taken together help to explain that while philosophy of science has developed with a more uniform intellectual orientation and a quite consensual institutional insertion notably in the United States and the United Kingdom in the 1960s and 1970s, philosophy of technology is heir to a much more heterogeneous lineage. Even when one looks at recent contributions to the field, it is striking to see how many of the academics who have made significant contributions to the philosophy of technology have received their university training outside the field.

These factors and others have combined to give rather a dispersed field. I am not the first to have pointed this out, with Val Dusek making a similar observation and putting it down, at least in part, to the disciplinary diversity of the constitutive elements of the philosophy of technology.

> The philosophy of technology involves the intimate interaction of a number of different fields of knowledge: philosophy of science, political and social philosophy, ethics, and some aesthetics and philosophy of religion. Specialists in ethics and political philosophy have rarely been deeply involved in the philosophy of science and vice versa.[20]

Nevertheless, as is the case for other disciplines in a similar situation, we can justifiably ask whether it is not the weakness of the identity of philosophy of technology as a field that is behind this disciplinary diversity rather than vice versa.

Starting in the 1970s, philosophy of science found its consensual foundations (in terms of both goals and methods) challenged by the rise of 'science studies,' which not only attacked many of the central tenets of logical-positivist philosophy of science, but also demanded a place for sociology and anthropology of science in the analysis of scientific practice and the constitution of scientific knowledge. Karl Popper and his followers, most famously Imre Lakatos, argued that sociological considerations were only useful for explaining why scientists had deviated from established scientific method, clinging to refuted theories or denying experimental evidence. The correct functioning of science required no such explanation because it was rational, underwriting an asymmetry in philosophy of science where the correct use of reason to arrive at the truth, and in particular its exemplification by the deployment of the scientific method, required no justification. Any irrational behavior, by contrast, had to be explained, usually, as we have said, by reference to sociological or, more commonly, psychological factors. Thus, philosophers like Lakatos proposed a division of intellectual labor, with philosophers of science explaining the results of the correct functioning of science and its progress toward the truth while sociology and psychology were to be called upon to explain any deviation from this path. In the manifesto of his 'strong program' published in 1976, David Bloor presented four tenets to serve as a basis for a new sociological approach to studying science. One of these four tenets was the principle of symmetry. An explanation of a scientific belief should be 'symmetrical in its style of explanation. The same types of cause would explain true and false beliefs.'[21] Leaving aside the thorny question of what type of account might be acceptable for a causal explanation of a scientist's beliefs in the strong program, we need to understand how this approach radically undermines the implicit conception of science in the philosophy of science, where truth serves as a guide for scientists and philosophers alike. The idea that both true and false beliefs should be explained in the same way challenged the status of science as a privileged means for knowing the world and undermined a comfortable relationship that philosophy of science had established with the sciences. The 1980s and 1990s saw the rise of a distinct field of 'science studies' where anthropological, historical and sociological tools were brought to bear to study the sciences. Accused of being relativist or at worst social constructivist, by the end of the twentieth century science studies represented a significant unruly dissident current of thought in the philosophy of the science.[22]

The upheaval brought about by the rise of science studies in the wake of the strong program did not spare the philosophy of technology. In the 1980s and 1990s, the critical approaches promoted by the adepts of science studies were mirrored by what we can term 'technology studies.' One particularly influential branch of this movement in the philosophy of technology was the Social Construction of Technology (SCOT) movement that adopted a stance clearly influenced by the strong program.

While this history of the philosophy of technology is not the same as that of the philosophy of science outlined above, we can note some similarities. In the 1950s, one could find certain philosophers proclaiming the neutrality of technology, as in this citation from the French author Pierre Ducassé.

> Technology is, by definition, perfectly and totally objective, because it can serve indifferently for completely contradictory ends; it is, in other words 'value neutral.'[23]

Nevertheless, although it is possible to find citations like this, the vision of technology as neutral was far from a consensual view. Ducassé himself was aware that others had doubts about this position, and he cites Jacques Ellul as someone who refused to accord this neutrality to technology. In the context of a much more ethically oriented philosophy of technology, Ellul maintained that it was artificial to separate any given technology from its use. Many histories of technology, however, even today limit their vision of a machine or other technological objects to a mechanical or technical response to a human need. Faced with the need to displace himself or herself rapidly over long distances, the technological response developed by humans has been the automobile. Going beyond this limited (and limiting) view of technology as a response to a social need takes us into the complex life of a technological object, and leads us to reflect on its social and political place and connotations. While taking these aspects into account remains contentious, widening our analysis to include the context in which a technology functions is necessary for opening up new debates concerning the place and functioning of technology in society. If we want to argue, for example, that the modern automobile represents and reinforces an individualistic approach to life and politics, we need to look further than the cars on the roads. We need to see how cars change patterns of living, patterns of sociability, and even patterns of political orientations.[24] The same is true of medical drugs. If we start from the supposition that such a drug is simply the appropriate technological response to a problem—a disease or infirmity—then we are already half way to an equally rationalist version of this drug's history.

Thus our own approach owes much to the SCOT program proposed by Trevor Pinch and Wiebe Bijker in the 1980s. Inspired, as we have said, by the Strong Program from the 1970s this movement explicitly challenged a rationalist (realist) approach in the philosophy of technology. [25] Bijker and Pinch took over the principle of symmetry directly from David Bloor and proposed explaining successful technologies in the same terms as failed ones (or vice versa). The key concept in SCOT, however, is 'interpretive flexibility,' the idea that the functions or meanings of technologies are not fixed but instead differ between and depend upon different social groups. This assertion amounts to a refusal to accept technological determinism understood in the sense that a technology introduced into society succeeds because it is an appropriate response (maybe even the correct response) to a given problem. For the proponents of SCOT, it is only in the process of closure of an episode and the stabilization of the 'winning' technology (with the elimination of the alternatives) that this choice is reinterpreted as the appropriate response and indeed that the function of the object is finally determined. This orientation toward the meaning given to technological artifacts by the relevant social groups is what makes the SCOT approach particularly interesting for my work in this book.

While the SCOT approach has informed my orientation toward the serum as technology, the structure of the book was inspired by a proposition made by Andrew Feenberg, in his 1999 publication, *Questioning Technology*. In a short passage, Feenberg lays out a schema that breaks the analysis of a technological object down into eight interrelated elements, grouped into two sets of four elements under the headings of primary and secondary instrumentalization. For Feenberg the process of primary instrumentalization covers the less social and more 'technical' side of the object considered in isolation, while the secondary aspects concern the integration of the object into technological systems and the social impact of the technology.[26] On the side of primary instrumentalization, Feenberg talks first of *de-worlding* as the separation of raw material from the natural world. In a logical, and for most objects, temporal progression de-worlding is followed by *reduction*, a transformation of the properties of the material in its naturally occurring state into those that make it useful in fulfilling the function for which it is ultimately intended as a technological object. The third element is that of *autonomization*, which involves turning the properties of the material to the advantage of the user. In the last aspect of this primary instrumentalization identified by Feenberg, he terms *positioning* and concerns the positioning of the object with respect to the conditions of production, distribution and sale.

Secondary instrumentalization, as we have already suggested opens up onto the more social aspects of the technological object. The first category, *systematization*, concerns the integration of the object into a technological system, and how its use combines with other objects within a network in the sense developed by Thomas Hugues in his analysis of large technical systems. The second element, *mediation*, Feenberg characterizes as 'ornamentation,' pointing to the ethical meaning of the object. Along with the other elements of secondary instrumentalization, vocation and initiative, these concepts proved to be particularly difficult to apply in this case as they are bound into a certain way of thinking about such objects that are specific to Feenberg's vision of technology as a domain for personal political struggle. For the sake of completeness, however, we can say that the third aspect of secondary instrumentalization, *vocation*, covers the effects the object has on those who use it. The last category Feenberg proposes, *initiative*, concerns the room for maneuver left to those who are generally seen as being subjugated to a given technology. While this approach via these eight categories proved helpful in laying out the initial argument, I found them ultimately too constraining for the analysis of the serum, particularly when it came to treating the social, professional and political meaning of the drug. Indeed, the last chapters aim to draw the contours of the French serum by examining the terms of its deployment in France, while the concepts of secondary instrumentalization limit us to considering the technology in the dynamic of its usage. For Feenberg, the object is defined by the attitude of the users (whether sanctioned or transgressive) to the technology and the effects that the technology in turn has on these users as well as the multiple opportunities opened up by this interaction. While these relations constitute part of the story of the introduction of serum in France, as we shall see in the closing chapters, the meaning for the drug was fashioned in a much wider arena than that of the action and retroaction of the serum on its users. In the end, Feenberg' schema proved to be a useful tool for thinking about this technological object, but, like Wittgenstein's conceptual ladder behind the *Tractactus*, it had to be laid aside in favor of a more open structure.[27]

THE STRUCTURE OF THE BOOK

The first chapter (Chapter 2) treats the obtention of the serum from the horses at the Pasteur Institute. This presentation of a concrete element in the production process already introduces us to an unexpected level of complexity, with the apparently straightforward process of drawing blood from horses being bound into a number of scientific and administrative systems (for producing and administering the toxin as well as managing the horses). This chapter is linked to Feenberg's concept of 'de-worlding' which describes an important element of any manufacturing process. Nevertheless, we underline how the complexity of the situation already leads us a certain distance away from the idealized philosophical examples usually chosen to illustrate the production of a technological object. With the raw material in hand, Chapter 3 takes us into the combination of formal and physical processes that transform the serum into a medical drug. Paying particular attention to the labeling of the product, we see what is implied by the series of tests undergone by the serum before it could be sent out for clinical use. The next chapter (Chapter 4) leads us deeper into an examination of the key notion of efficacy, exploring the means for establishing that a drug is effective against the disease it is used to treat. Looking at how efficacy is constructed ties into a familiar debate in the philosophy of science, as what lies behind this analysis is the issue of the reality of the drug's effect. Putting to one side the 'objective' question of whether the drug worked or not, we choose to look at the mechanisms in play in the construction of the proof or perception of efficacy. Although, as I have already explained, my approach is informed by the more constructivist trends in the philosophy of technology, I remain agnostic on the fundamental issue; leaving, as I have said, the ontological question of the drug's effect aside and examining the arguments that were made about it, the aim is to assess their form rather than their merit.

Chapter 5 diverts attention away from the serum in favor of the disease it was used to treat: diphtheria. The evolving diagnosis and identity of the disease at the turn of the century was intimately tied to the development of serotherapy at several levels. Here, we see the importance that bacteriology was starting to assume in France. The French institution most intimately associated with bacteriology a century ago, as it still is today, was the Pasteur Institute, and Chapter 6 looks at how this Institute organized the production of serum for France, paying particular attention to how this enterprise was financed. Having established the strong links between the Pasteur Institute and the serum, the next chapter (Chapter 7) goes on to look at the image of diphtheria and the serum in France, emphasizing how the treatment bound together children, women and the medical profession around what was perceived as a new miracle drug. The last chapter before the conclusion turns to the political context of serum production in France under the Third Republic. Here we consider the legislation that was hurriedly put into place to cover this drug, before reflecting on the situation outside Paris. Looking more closely at what happened in Lyon and Nancy, we see how local initiatives worked against the centralized monopoly of the Pasteur Institute, freeing up resources in provincial towns for the promotion of microbiology as well as the local provision of serum. Although less clearly elaborated than the claim about French serum, the argument underlying this final chapter is that not all

French serum was necessarily the same. We close, therefore, with the suggestion that serum from Nancy or Le Havre, was not the same as serum from Paris or Lille.

As the book advances, the presentation of the serum leads us progressively further away from the taxonomy proposed by Feenberg. In the end, the reflection on how the social and political meaning of the drug informs the object itself is the richest part of the book's contribution to the philosophy of technology. While there is nothing original about the idea that technological choice and development are influenced by social and political considerations, here we are arguing that the object itself is informed by the place it assumes in society.[28] Thus, we begin to see more clearly how the French serum is constructed differently from serum in neighboring countries. In the end, the problem we raised—that medical drugs do not resemble the typical examples deployed in the philosophy of technology—reveals its positive side. The implication of the social and political context in the construction of the drug as object can help us to think more clearly about this aspect for other objects where an analysis of the mechanical operation too easily distracts us from these issues.

THE PHILOSOPHICAL ORIENTATION OF THIS STUDY

On a more personal note, I would like to explain why this book looks neither like a typical contribution to the philosophy of technology nor like a typical monograph in the history of medicine. Initially trained in the philosophy of science, during my doctoral studies I turned toward the history of science.[29] Throughout my subsequent career, I have always been interested in the philosophical questions raised by the sciences, although pursuing more historical analyses. Exploring the history of pharmacy has led me to think about the place of this discipline among the sciences, and how to understand its hybrid nature as being always an applied science as much as a theoretical one. In this respect pharmacy might be a richer exemplar of modern science than the idealized versions of theoretical physics that have traditionally served as the standard models for philosophers. Another element that arose from this reflection about the hybrid nature of pharmacy was the idea that the philosophy of technology might provide a key to better understanding the history of pharmacy than the philosophy of science.

Turning once more to the philosophy of technology, we see that its proponents have tended to be more engaged (both politically and socially) than their counterparts in the philosophy of science. Challenges to the value of modern technology have been present in this area since its beginning, with Jacques Ellul and Ivan Illich, the leading figures in the critical interrogation of technology. The question of whether technology is the means to liberate humans from labor and other constraints or the means to control their thought and actions was posed early on and continues to be asked, notably with respect to information and communication technologies. Although I do not develop it here, this line of questioning is evidently pertinent to medical drugs that, under the guise of saving or prolonging human life, have succeeded in infiltrating every aspect of human life, being used to modulate our moods, sleeping patterns, aging and sexuality. Thus, this passage via pharmacy from philosophy of science to medical drugs has opened up new and interesting perspectives that I never imagined as a student. This work is an attempt to profit from this reflection by bringing a philosophical reflection to bear on a historical case that I have had the opportunity to explore in some depth. I hope that this work can serve as a useful model for others who want to think historically about issues in the philosophy of science, or more specifically the philosophy of technology.

SEROTHERAPY AS MEDICAL DRUG

To close this introduction, I want to say a few words about why I have chosen serotherapy, and, in particular, serotherapy in France for this study as well as signaling certain elements that will not be treated. Following a collaboration on a German project comparing serum production in France and in Germany, [30] I have now been studying this medical innovation for almost a decade, although principally focused on its production and use in France. There are many possible ways to present this material, and certain choices had to be made. The most evident is limiting the study to France and not considering the situation in other European countries, notably Germany, Britain, Italy, Switzerland, Spain and Norway. As I have already suggested, the choice of France allows me to develop a position that would be much more difficult to argue at the level of a European comparison, even though it would be just as valid. I have also limited my analysis to the therapeutic use of the serum (its use on people considered to be suffering from diphtheria), and have left its prophylactic use to one side. While the serum was used as a preventive measure like a vaccine, in France this use was marginal. There were no large-scale campaigns of vaccination against diphtheria using the serum, and, in particular, there were no high-profile accidents implicating this practice like the Langerhans case in Germany.[31]

While the present study explores the case of serotherapy as a treatment for diphtheria, I believe that this approach could be usefully employed to analyze other medical drugs. Of course certain features, notably the rich national meaning assumed by serotherapy in France at the end of the nineteenth century, would not be found in such a clear form in other cases. French serum is, therefore, both unique and a model for thinking about medical drugs as technological objects.

NOTES

1. For an example of this classic conception in the philosophy of science where the world is given as true or false units of sense data, see Rudolf Carnap, *Der Logische aufbau der Welt*. (Berlin, Schlachtensee Welkreis-Verlag, 1928). In a sense Robert Merton's principle of 'universalism' is an extension of this idea onto sociological ground, because the idea that the characteristics of the scientist should play no role in the appreciation of his or her scientific theory is premised on the principle that the theory is true or false independently of the community of scientists. Robert Merton, 'The Normative Structure of Science' in *The Sociology of Science: Theoretical and Empirical Investigations*, (Chicago: University of Chicago Press, 1979) pp. 267–78, originally published in 1942.

2. Except, of course, to cast aspersions on the quality of the product itself, but this kind of argument is generally reserved for the combat between name brands and generic products rather than criticisms of clinical trials.

3. For an interesting treatment of the dissemination of the use of the thermometer in the clinic in Germany, see Volker Hess, *Der wohltemperierte Mensch: Wissenschaft und Alltag des Fiebermessens (1850–1900)* (Frankfurt am Main: Campus Verlag, 2000).

4. These articles are often published in scientific journals; see, Abdallah Fayssoil 'René Laennec (1781–1826) and the Invention of the Stethoscope.' *The American Journal of Cardiology* 104, n° 5 (2009): 743–4 or Daniel H. Robinson and Alexander H. Toledo. 'Historical Development of Modern Anesthesia.' *Journal of Investigative Surgery: The Official Journal of the Academy of Surgical Research* 25, n° 3 (2012): 141–9.

5. Joel D. Howell, *Technology in the Hospital: Transforming Patient Care in the Early Twentieth Century* (Baltimore: The Johns Hopkins University Press, 1996). More recent explorations of medical technologies have tended to focus on the laboratory rather than the clinic, for example Tricia Close-Koenig, 'Betwixt and Between. Production and Commodification of Knowledge in a Medical School Pathological Anatomy Laboratory, Strasbourg (mid-nineteenth Century to 1939)' (Phd Thesis, University of Strasbourg, 2011).

6. Thomas Schlich, *The Origins of Organ Transplantation: Surgery and Laboratory Science, 1880–1930* (Rochester: University of Rochester Press, 2010) Carsten Timmermann and Julie Anderson (eds), *Devices and designs: medical technologies in historical perspective*. (Houndmills: Palgrave Macmillan, 2006).

7. Images of such deep fermentors from the Merck archives can be seen on the website, 'http://herbarium.usu.edu' under 'fun facts about fungi' on the penicillin page (accessed July 14, 2016)

8. For a history of the rise of the pharmaceutical industry in France, see Sophie Chauveau, *L'Invention pharmaceutique: la pharmacie française entre l'état et la société au XXe siècle* (Paris: Sanofi-Synthélabo, 1999).

9. This is the version of the penicillin story we get in Ruth Cowan's book on technology in America, for example, where she treats this antibiotic and the birth-control pill as technological items. Ruth Schwartz Cowan, *A Social History of American Technology* (Oxford: Oxford University Press, 1997), pp. 310–8.

10. Anne Rasmussen, 'Les enjeux d'une histoire des formes pharmaceutiques : La galénique, l'officine et l'industrie (XIXe – début XXe siècle),' *Entreprises et histoire*, n° 36, 2 (2004), 12–28.

11. Jeremy Greene, *Prescribing by Numbers: Drugs and the Definition of Disease* (Baltimore: The Johns Hopkins University Press, 2006), p. 130

12. For a brief overview of the standardization of drugs, see the introduction to Christoph Gradmann and Jonathan Simon (eds), *Evaluating and Standardizing Therapeutic Agents, 1890–1950*. (Basingstoke: Palgrave Macmillan, 2010).

13. Joseph C. Pitt, *Doing Philosophy of Technology: Essays in a Pragmatist Spirit* (Dordrecht: Springer, 2011).

14. Carl Mitcham, *Thinking through Technology : The Path between Engineering and Philosophy* (Chicago: University of Chicago Press, 1994), p. 161.

15. An early example in this vein was Paul de Kruif, *Microbe Hunters* (New York: Kessinger Publishing, 1926), but the trend continues with François Chast, *Histoire contemporaine des médicaments* (Paris: La Découverte, 2002) constituting a more recent French contribution to this genre.

16. See, for example, Nicolas Rasmussen, *On Speed: The Many Lives of Amphetamine* (New York: NYU Press, 2009) and Elizabeth Siegel Watkins, *On the Pill: A Social History of Oral Contraceptives, 1950–1970* (Baltimore: Johns Hopkins University Press, 2001).

17. This, of course, puts to one side the French tradition of philosophy of science, where one would cite Bachelard, Canguilhem and Koyré. Dominique Lecourt makes a good attempt at presenting both traditions in his introduction to philosophy of science; Dominique Lecourt, *La philosophie des sciences* (Paris: Presses Universitaires de France, 2010).

18. Another foundational text that is often cited is Ernst Kapp, *Grundlinien einer Philosophie der Technik: zur Entstehungsgeschichte der Cultur aus neuen Gesichtspunkten* (Braunschweig: G. Westermann, 1877).

19. While the title Philosophy of Science and Technology is not uncommon for graduate programs or academic departments, I have been unable to find a program that bears the title Philosophy of Technology and Science.

20. Val Dusek, *Philosophy of Technology: an Introduction* (Oxford: Blackwell, 2006).

21. David Bloor, *Knowledge and Social Imagery*. (London: Routledge & Kegan Paul, 1976), p. 7.

22. For a good overview of the developments in this area, see David Hess, *Science studies: An advanced introduction*. (New York: New York University Press, 1997).

23. Elle [la technique] est, par définition, d'une parfaite et totale objectivité, puisqu'elle peut servir indifféremment les fins les plus contradictoires : elle est, dit-on encore neutre à la valeur.' Pierre Ducassé, *Les techniques et le philosophe*. (Paris: Presses Universitaires de France, 1958), p. 7.

24. A study of the car in the US was crucial in Illich's conception of the notion of counterproductivity, arguing that cars had the opposite function to the one imputed to them by technological rationalists: Ivan Illich, *Energy and Equity* (New York: Marion Boyars, 1974).

25. Trevor Pinch and Wiebe Bijker, 'The Social Construction of Facts and Artefacts: Or How the Sociology of Science and the Sociology of Technology Might Benefit Each Other,' *Social Studies of Science*, 14 (1984), 399–441.

26. Andrew Feenberg, *Questioning Technology* (London: Routledge, 1999), pp. 202–7.

27. Ludwig Wittgenstein, *Tractatus Logico-Philosophicus*, transl. C. K. Ogden (London: Kegan Paul, Trench, Trubner & Co, 1922), p. 90 (6. 54). 'My propositions are elucidatory in this way: he who understands me finally recognizes them as senseless, when he has climbed out through them, on them, over them. (He must so to speak throw away the ladder, after he has climbed up on it.)'

28. The best-known example of political influence on technological decisions is that of the height of bridges on the freeways to Long Island, restricting access to the working class by bus. See, Langdon Winner 'Do Artifacts Have Politics?' in *The Whale and the Reactor: A Search for Limits in an Age of High Technology*, edited by Langdon Winner, 19–39. Chicago: Chicago University Press, 1986.

29. This thesis has since been published as a book: Jonathan Simon, *Chemistry, Pharmacy and Revolution*. (Aldershot: Ashgate, 2005).

30. The project entitled 'The Industrialisation of Experimental Knowledge' was run by Volker Hess and financed by the German Research Foundation (DFG HE 2220/4–1 & 2).

31. In 1896, Ernst Langerhans, the son of a prominent German pathologist died after a prophylactic injection of serum. The ensuing investigation was the subject of considerable media attention. See, Axel Hüntelmann, 'The Anti-Diphtheria Serum and the Case of Langerhans.' *Medizin, Gesellschaft, und Geschichte: Jahrbuch des Instituts für Geschichte der Medizin der Robert Bosch Stiftung* 24 (2005): 71–104.

Chapter 2

Blood

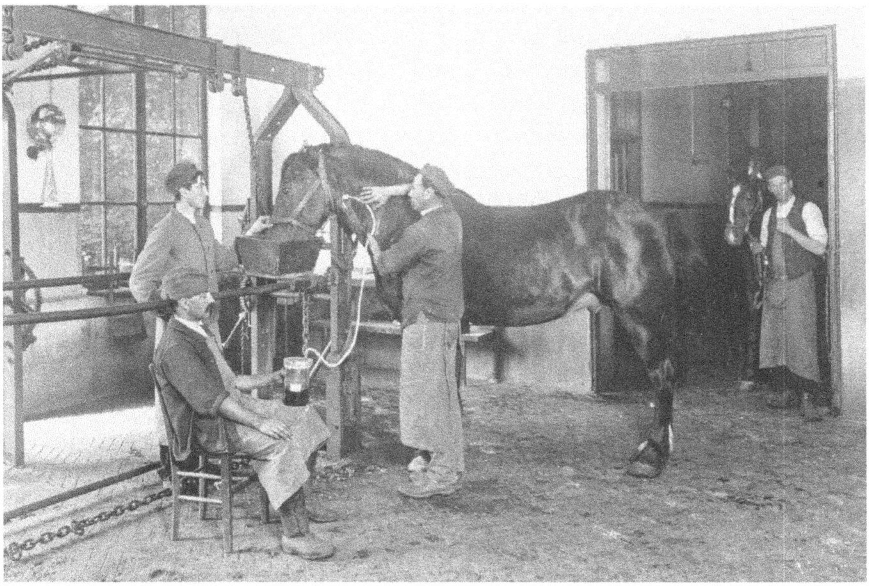

Figure 2.1 Bleeding a horse at the Pasteur Institut, Garches, circa 1910. © Institut Pasteur—Musée Pasteur.

In Goethe's version of *Faust*, Mephisto refuses to accept Faust's word of honor as sufficient guarantee for the contract on his soul. While any piece of paper will do for drawing up the contract, the devil's envoy insists that Faust seal the pact with a drop of his own blood. For, as Mephisto explains, 'blood is quite a special liquid.'[1] Emil Behring and Shibasaburo Kitasato, two researchers working at Robert Koch's Institute for Infectious Disease in Berlin, published their seminal paper on the potential of acquired immunity as the basis for a treatment for infectious disease in December 1890 and ended the article by quoting this well-known line from Goethe, thereby evoking the rich cultural significance of blood.[2] But Behring and Kitasato were citing Goethe in the context of a very specific transformation of this biological material, with the intervention they described in the article inscribing animal blood in a new era of therapy. Their experiments involved immunizing rabbits against tetanus by inoculation with in vitro cultures of the microbe responsible for the disease. They then injected the blood serum (the part of the blood left after the red blood corpuscles had been separated out from the rest) from these immunized rabbits into mice that they subsequently infected with tetanus. The researchers found that while the mice that had received the serum were unaffected by a lethal dose of tetanus, the control mice that had not received the serum were all killed by it. This is how Behring and Kitasato demonstrated that the immunity against the disease could be transferred from one animal to another via the serum. They, of course, made sure that the serum of non-immunized animals did not have the same prophylactic properties and went on to demonstrate the capacity of serum from immunized animals to kill the tetanus bacilli in vitro. Furthermore, the protection offered by the serum was quite specific, with serum from an animal immunized against diphtheria, for example, offering no protection against tetanus but preventing the ill effects of infection with diphtheria. While this was not the first time that scientists had proposed the idea of using blood in the treatment of a disease, the approach presented in this pioneering article nevertheless formed the basis for a radically new form of treatment that came to be known as serotherapy.[3]

Behring and Kitasato explicitly evoked the application of the principle of serotherapy to the treatment of both tetanus and diphtheria in humans in their 1890 publication, and it would take only a year for the German researchers to pass from this preliminary work in the immunization of animals to the first experimental use of serum to treat diphtheria in a child. The research that led to this first diphtheria serum was undertaken by Behring in collaboration with Erich Wernicke, a friend who was also a colleague at Robert Koch's institute. Although clearly pioneers in this research, Behring and Wernicke were not alone in trying to develop this therapy for large-scale use, with competition in Berlin from Hans Aronson and in Paris from Emile Roux. When Behring became disabled by several bouts of depression, Wernicke, who had almost died from diphtheria at the age of 17, dedicated himself to finding a technique that worked. After the Institute's only ram died following a massive dose of virulent diphtheria culture, Wernicke personally paid for three more wethers (castrated rams) that he and his fiancée housed and fed. These wethers were immunized against diphtheria using a technique of graduated exposure to progressively increasing volumes of the microbe responsible for the disease. In December 1891, one year after the publication by Kitasato and Behring, and thanks to the help of Paul Geissler, Wernicke successfully treated a child at the Bergmannsche Clinic in Berlin using a massive fifty cubic centimeters of serum taken from one of his wethers.[4]

This initial success was followed by the switch to horses as the animal of choice and some disappointing demonstrations of the therapeutic activity of the serum in Berlin. Nevertheless, Behring managed to overcome the reigning skepticism concerning this new therapy and in the spring of 1893 negotiated a partnership with the chemical manufacturer Meister, Lucius and Brüning in Hoechst. Considerable investment by the company allowed a scaling up of serum production to levels where it could be made available as a commercial product, and the so-called 'Behring serum' first went on sale in August 1893.[5] As we shall see in more detail in what follows, the research at the Pasteur Institute in France ran over a year behind this pioneering German work, with large-scale serum production only put into place in Paris at the very beginning of 1895.

TAKING BLOOD FROM HORSES

In Feenberg's schema, when considering primary instrumentalization, the first step in the transformation of a natural object is its decontextualization or 'de-worlding.'[6] As a prerequisite for its human use, the material intended for the construction of the object needs first to be extracted from its natural environment and therefore from a network of relationships that bind it to this original context. This intervention serves to release (or constitute) the technological potential of the object as something quite distinct from its function in its natural environment.

The example that is often given is of a length of wood turned into an axe handle. After felling a tree, a piece of wood has to be carved into the appropriate shape for use. What was part of the tree becomes a length of wood in a particular form that bears no resemblance to the original living organism in terms of either form or function. This piece of wood is now ready to be integrated into the technological object that is the axe.

On this model, then, the first thing we need to consider is how blood, a naturally occurring substance, came to be removed from its original context allowing it subsequently to be mobilized as a medical drug. To simplify the analysis, we will consider only the mature production process using horses, and not the various experimental stages that mobilized guinea pigs, dogs and rams, among other animals. Even limited to a single species, however, the preparation of the animal and the obtention of the blood serum are not as straightforward as they may at first appear. As will become clear, even before the bleeding process blood was transformed through a sophisticated technological intervention on the horses, an intervention itself dependent on a series of microbial manipulations.

The blood in a horse, or in any other mammal for that matter, performs numerous biological functions. The role of red blood cells in distributing oxygen from the lungs throughout the body is usually the first to be presented in biology classes, but blood performs other roles as well, prominent among them is the immunological function of the white blood cells. While this immunological function is evidently important and is directly related to serotherapy, I do not want to explore the biological function of blood any further, beyond noting the vital importance of blood for horses. Like other vertebrates, horses cannot live without their blood although they can lose a significant amount of it without dying and can replace lost blood relatively quickly.[7] The vital nature of blood, as well as its unique capacity to regenerate, have contributed to its special status in human society; for many Christians, for example, wine is converted into blood by the miraculous act of consecration during the sacrament, and the evacuation of blood is a central element in the slaughter of animals for Jews and Moslems alike.[8] As I suggested at the beginning of this chapter, blood is particularly rich in its significance and this in large part because of its ritual use. In turn, the importance that blood has assumed in many rituals can only be explained by reference to its symbolic status. Thus, paradoxically, while the bleeding of an animal literally removes the blood from its original corporal context where it performs a number of vital functions, the process of bleeding can amplify the significance of the material. The blood that Lady Macbeth cannot wash off her hands or the blood that splashed on the face of the witness to a murder in a film no longer serves to keep someone alive, but is highly significant in modern culture. The mode of production of the serum served to reduce this significance to a minimum. The parallel can be drawn with large-scale abattoirs where the passage of huge numbers of animals and the technological routinization of their slaughter de-naturalizes them, transforming them—and in the process their blood as well—into little more than raw material for processed food. Under these conditions, the death of a cow is no longer seen as a death but has been transformed into a preliminary step in the beef manufacturing process. Likewise, the daily bleedings at the Pasteur Institute's serum manufacturing facilities were not treated as sacrificial rites but were organized following an industrial mode of production. This being said, the distinction between blood and serum as a therapeutic agent was inscribed not only in the day-to-day production of the serum, but also in the prior preparation of the horses that lay behind this production. To make this clearer, we will approach the multifacetted process of serum production in stages.

To obtain blood serum from any warm-blooded animal, you first need to bleed the animal and then separate out the red blood cells. In the manufacture of therapeutic sera, the blood was removed from an animal through a vein using a trocar that could be attached to a tube leading to a receiver. Thus the blood was taken from the living animal using a practice that can be observed with any blood donation operation. The serum was then obtained from the blood by letting the blood clot naturally and separating the serum from the congealed red blood cells. While at the Pasteur Institute the blood was just left to stand, other serum producers used centrifugation to speed up the process, but the principle remained the same. The serum was then distributed into individual phials, standardly containing a volume of 20 or 10 cubic centimeters. This process of bleeding, separation and distribution quite literally produced the serum as a material available for use starting from an organic substance found within a living animal, but we have not yet touched on the essential interventions on the host animal made prior to the bleeding and coagulation. The blood serum of a normal horse was considered ineffective against diphtheria. All the horses that were bled to produce the anti-diphtheria serum, whether at Hoechst in Germany or at the Pasteur Institute's various facilities in Paris, were immunized against diphtheria prior to the bleeding. Here, then, there is an important difference from the case in which a tree is cut down and then carved to obtain the wood for an axe handle (at least in the rare case where the tree has grown wild in a forest), as the prior intervention on the living organism is constitutive of the technological object in question. In this case, the horse itself had been artificially transformed—in a sense 'de-naturalized'—even before being bled.

To further complicate matters, we want to insist on the fact that this prior transformation of the horse has its own history as an innovative scientific technique. Different methods for immunizing the horses were tested before the producers settled on an approach that gave reliable results with the least perceptible or foreseeable risk, but even then in-house researchers continued to vary the parameters of the process in order to improve yields. The first immunizations were achieved using in vitro cultures of the pathogenic bacteria, but this technique soon ceded its place to an alternative route for immunization using the toxin produced by the microbes rather than the microbes themselves.[9] The production of this toxin for use in the immunization process demanded its own technological system, which developed alongside serum production. The first down-to-earth goal was to administer the toxin to the horse without killing it, and, having succeeded in this preliminary step, the subsidiary aim was to obtain as high a level of immunization as possible. Globally, the strategy was to start with small doses of the toxin (often treated with a chemical disinfectant to reduce the toxicity even further) and gradually to increase the quantities until the immunizing power of the serum—as determined by tests of immunizing power carried out on guinea pigs—was at its maximum. In order to immunize the horses, however, the serum manufacturers needed a regular supply of predictably potent toxin, which meant cultivating particular strains of the living microbes that produced it. Samples of the diphtheria bacillus were regularly collected from dead and dying children and then tested experimentally in the search for an appropriate strain. We can, therefore, also consider the diphtheria toxin used to immunize the horses as itself a technological object produced from a living system.[10] Although we will not pursue this line of argument, it is clear that it sets us on a potentially long regressive path of such objects, passing from the bacteria to the children from whom they were isolated. Limiting our analysis to the toxin, however, we can see the importance it assumed in the production of serum by considering the work of Louis Martin who took charge of the day-to-day running of the facilities at the Pasteur Institute starting at the end of 1894.

Like Emile Roux, the head of serum production at the Pasteur Institute, Louis Martin was a physician. Although still a medical student when he replaced Alexandre Yersin as Roux's assistant at the Institute in 1893, Martin went on to qualify as a doctor in 1897, writing a thesis entitled 'The Production of Diphtheria Toxin' (*Production de la toxine diphtérique*). Here, he presented the results of over two years of experience and research in the production of diphtheria serum. As he explains it, the goal of his research was to determine how to produce the greatest amount of toxin in the shortest time. For this, he studied a range of parameters that entered into play, including the nature of the culture medium (its acidity, the passage of air and its composition), the strain of the bacteria and the physical conditions in which they were cultured. He concluded that it was best to keep the medium alkaline and proposed a detailed recipe for the optimal culture medium. This mixture was composed of macerated (fresh) veal to which was added 'peptonized' water, prepared by boiling stomachs of pigs. The resulting 'bouillon' was heated to 70 degrees and then filtered before introducing the bacteria. Working from a panel of eight different strains (each originating from a sample taken from a different patient infected with diphtheria), Martin obtained the best results with the No. 8 bacillus provided by the American microbiologists William Park and Anna Williams. In an appendix to his thesis Louis Martin also presented his protocol for the filtration of the culture to give the toxin in solution that would be used for immunizing the horses. Filtering the bacterial culture through a porcelain Chamberland filter under vacuum gave a solution of the toxin free from the pathogenic microbe.

Martin concluded his thesis with an explanation of the practical pay-off of his research. He claimed that through his experiments he had succeeded in multiplying the toxic strength of the toxin tenfold and that the use of this toxin for immunization led to a serum with twice as much immunizing power as before.[11]

This digression through the process of toxin production makes it clear how the blood in the horses used for serum production was not a 'natural' organic raw material but was already the product of elaborate human-technological intervention. Furthermore, this intervention involved the cultivation of toxin and experimenting with different techniques of immunization both of which had their own histories. The potency of the toxin was guaranteed by a series of experiments and controls governing its production, purification and use, and, as we saw with the example of Louis Martin's research into toxin production, all these processes were subject to change over time. Thus, the conditioning of the horses prior to their bleeding is premised on a technological engagement tied into the nascent science of microbiology.[12]

While the immunization process represents the beginning of the active intervention on the horses, in order to be integrated into the production process the animals were also removed from the world in a different sense. Even before receiving their first injection with the toxin, the horses had passed through a selection process. While the criteria were not very stringent, they still limited the choice to a minority of the available animals. In a book on serotherapy, Georges Lemière described the criteria adopted by the Pasteur Institute.

> Which horses are chosen to prepare the antitoxic serum? It is necessary to select horses that are still young, 8 to 10 years old maximum, as they need to eat well, ones that have no constitutional illness, and, as far as is possible, that have never previously suffered from an infectious disease, because this would render them more sensitive to the action of the toxin.[13]

It was Edmond Nocard, a professor at the veterinary school in Alfort and a close collaborator in the development of serum production at the Pasteur Institute, who was in charge of screening the horses. Nocard had entered Louis Pasteur's laboratory as an assistant in 1880, working alongside Emile Roux as an assistant in Pasteur's anthrax research. By the 1890s he had established himself as a leading figure in microbiology in France, one of a handful of fully fledged Pastorians who was not employed directly at the Institute. Using his knowledge in microbiology Nocard had developed a test for glanders but otherwise he was limited, like other veterinarians of the period, to the most accessible symptoms for detecting the presence of diseases in the horses. Thus, the selection was restricted to considerations such as age, general physical condition and the owner's testimony concerning the horse's health. Whatever the details, Roux was grateful for Nocard's support, as his own speciality was managing microorganisms and not large animals. With the scale of production of serum increasing, Roux needed all the help he could get from professional veterinarians, and Nocard provided a personal link to this professional group. Roux returned to this point on the occasion of the inauguration of a memorial to Nocard at the veterinary school.

> When serotherapy was introduced, we would never have been able to install a service capable of responding to the legitimate impatience of the public so promptly without Nocard. His qualities as an organizer and leader, and his experimental skill saved us in this affair. The laboratory at Alfort became a kind of branch of the Pasteur Institute: here, Nocard prepared the serum and taught the young veterinarians who later became our precious collaborators, animated by the spirit of their master.[14]

Selected for this quite novel use as the producers of medical drugs, the horses were removed from their daily work of pulling cabs, gun carriages or carts (or even, occasionally, taken from racing stables, as we shall see in Chapter 6), and were placed in a new environment where they could be injected with toxin, monitored and made readily available for bleeding. At first, when there were only a few, the horses were kept in or near the Pasteur Institute in Paris, with the production process centered on this site.[15] As the number of horses increased, however, they were moved to a specialized facility at Garches, outside Paris.[16] Here, the horses gave up their names (if they had ever had one) in favor of a number, which was branded onto one of their front hooves. As these numbers only went as high as 99, the horses were either branded on their left or their right hoof, allowing the administration to follow almost two hundred animals with a suffix of either G (for gauche—left) or D (droite—right).

The horses were now managed as administrative units as in any other production facility. Thus, each one had its own entries or even pages in a series of registers, tracking the injections with toxin, the measured immunizing power of the serum produced by the animal, as well as all the bleedings it was subject to. The horses were integrated into groups that were bled and immunized on the same shift, although a bleeding with a low immunization power would mean the horse being removed from its usual group. If attempts to re-establish its immunity failed, the horse would be disposed of definitively.

Overall, we can characterize the group of procedures described above (selection of horses, immunization and bleeding) as the means of 'de-worlding' the serum. But we can also see that the process is already more complex than the idea as it is presented by Andrew Feenberg. When a person, or group of people, aims to make an axe handle from a tree, the tree is cut down and the wood stripped and fashioned into the desired form. At the end of this process, the axe handle while made from the wood of a tree is no longer a tree. It is this distance that Feenberg invites us to consider, and the processes involved in removing the material from its natural context, the first step in making it useful, rather than simply exploiting some inherent utility. This approach has the advantage of avoiding the Aristotelian temptation of considering technology (*techne*) as essentially imitative of a natural means to the same end.[17]

But with serum we are not in the same configuration as with the axe handle. The horses used for serum production had already been removed from their original context (for the majority of them as working animals, well integrated into the functioning of a modern late nineteenth-century city like Paris) in order to serve as production units for the medical drug. For this, they underwent a very specific technical intervention that transformed their bodies. This intervention suggests that we need to consider these horses as technological objects in their own right, just as we were initially thinking of serum in these terms. While their principal function is certainly redefined by their transfer from 'civil' life to the Pasteur Institute, they remain recognizably horses, fed and groomed by a specialized staff. Furthermore, the horses were not put to use for treating disease directly, and so it might be more pertinent to consider them as tools or production units rather than as objects comparable to the serum.[18] The artificiality of these horses both in terms of their life at Garches and the interventions made on them in order to produce the serum might well warrant further attention, but, having signaled these different levels of complexity, I nevertheless want to return my attention to the serum itself.

PACKAGING THE SERUM

The bleeding and separation of serum from the blood were followed by its conditioning; the final packaging before the product could leave the Pasteur Institute. Initially, the distribution of the serum was limited to the Parisian hospitals as well as to doctors who came and knocked at the door of Roux's laboratory in Paris. Starting in January 1895, however, the phials of serum were distributed all over France through an elaborate but largely ad hoc network that we will discuss later. The Pasteur Institute even introduced a system for ordering by telegraph to help deal with the size and the scope of demand. Thus, this final step in the physical extraction and preparation of the serum required putting it in phials ready for injection then packaging them for dispatch first within Paris and later all across France. It should be noted that in moving from the bleeding to the bottling we have skipped over an important stage in the process, the evaluation of the immunization power of the serum, but we will cover this in detail in the next chapter.

At the beginning, the Pasteur Institute produced the anti-diphtheria serum for retail in volumes of 20 cubic centimeters. This contrasted with the offer from its German counterparts like Hoechst and Schering who proposed different strengths of serum in 10 and 20 cubic-centimeter doses. With little competition on the French market,[19] the Pasteur Institute had no particular incentive to diversify its offer. Nevertheless, it seems that within a year the standard dose had been reduced to a 10 cc format, giving doctors more options in terms of the quantity of serum administered to the patients. Whether 20 or 10 cubic centimeters, the uniformity of the doses offered by the Pasteur Institute simplified this final stage of preparation before the product left the premises.

The Pasteur Institute was less than ten years old when it started manufacturing the serum against diphtheria. While part of the new buildings were used to produce the vaccine for the treatment of rabies, the facilities—built thanks to an international subscription for an institute for rabies treatment, microbiology teaching and research—were mainly given over to research laboratories. In order to accommodate the serum production, which would be on a much larger scale than the rabies vaccine, Emile Roux organized the transfer of the horses to a new location at Garches (also known as Villeneuve l'Etang or Marnes-la-Coquette), outside Paris. But he also dedicated a part of the research space in the Institute in Paris to the serotherapy project, refitting certain rooms for bottling and dispatching the serum. Thus, the large flasks of serum, that contained the serum from one bleeding (around 3 liters each), were brought from Garches to Paris, where the precious liquid was decanted into the phials that, once sealed, could be used for treatment. The refurbishment of the Paris site was probably finished at the end of 1894, as in October of that year it was still in the planning stage.

> At the Pasteur Institute they will make do with fitting out a large laboratory on the first floor of the building—formerly reserved for cages of rabbits—for the preparation and dispatching of the vaccine [sic]. Under the permanent direction of M. Roux, two doctors will be responsible for the preparation of the serum, which requires many precautions and a great deal of care.[20]

These spacious, well-lit rooms became the part of the overall process of serum production that most resembled industrial manufacture of the time, at least in appearance. This resemblance was particularly striking in two respects; the use of dedicated machines and the reliance on women to perform the repetitive precision tasks involved in these final steps of serum production.

In this pair of photographs from the early part of the twentieth century (Figure 2.2) we can see two women at work at the Pasteur Institute in these final stages of production. The woman in the foreground is decanting the serum into phials using a machine specifically designed by Emile Roux for dispensing the 20 cubic centimeter (and later 10cc) doses. The woman presses on a foot pedal to release the required volume of serum into the small bottles she is holding at the end of the piping that emerges from the bottom of

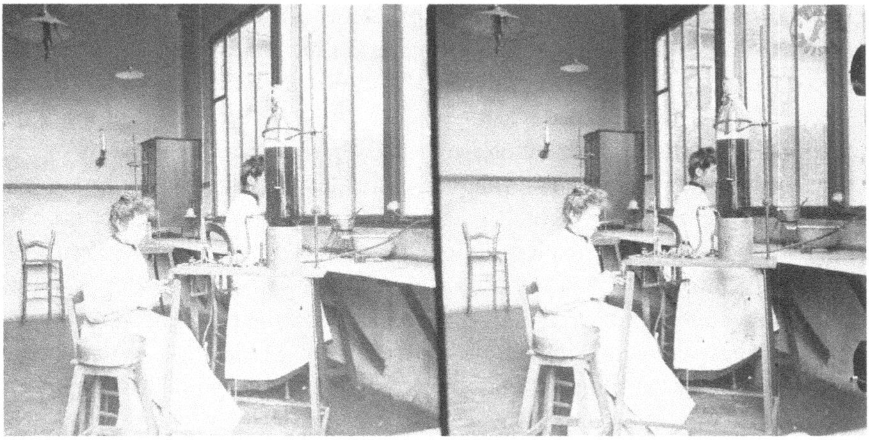

Figure 2.2 Photograph of two women preparing phials of serum at the Pasteur Institute, circa 1910. Possibly for a stereoscopic picture. © Institut Pasteur - Musée Pasteur

the large bottle. The design of Roux's machine and the position adopted by its operators echo those associated with sewing machines as well as some early versions of the typewriter. The woman's hair is tied up to keep it free of the working parts of the machine and she is wearing white overalls to protect her clothes. Whether operating a sewing machine in a factory, working for a typing pool or dispensing serum into phials, women had to carefully coordinate the movement of their hands and feet in this task, repeating the same series of movements thousands of times a day. While the public, high-profile research side of the Pasteur Institute was uniquely populated by men, the production side associated with serotherapy relied on the labor of women.

Before concluding this reflection on the de-worlding of serum, I want to briefly consider the geography of this multistep process, in particular its distribution across the different types of physical sites. The stables at Marnes-la-Coquette (Garches), formerly home to Napoléon-Bonaparte's élite cavalry squadron the *cent-gardes*, constituted a rural and essentially male domain. Stable boys and veterinary staff looked after the horses and ensured that they followed the production regime imposed from above.[21] After being separated from the clotted red blood cells, the serum was then physically moved (probably taking advantage of the passage of the railway line through the grounds of the domain) to the Pasteur Institute in Paris. Here a female staff prepared it for distribution in labeled injectable units as we just saw. The Pasteur Institute organized the production process into hierarchical and gendered units similar to a range of other industrial manufacturing systems from the end of the nineteenth century in France.[22]

What appeared at first to be a simple preliminary step of taking the blood from the horse (taking a natural product, albeit a symbolically highly charged one, and rendering it artificial and independent) turns out to be much more complex. A series of interventions rendered the horses artificial using an experimentally produced and perfected diphtheria toxin.

It would perhaps be more accurate to talk of the re-alignment of a highly technologized world. The elements of what we will see later in terms of the constitutive expertise and control that guarantee the quality of this mass-produced drug were there from the beginning of the production process. On another level, the horse itself was integrated into a productive system that configured the serum. As is the case with nearly all modern drugs, these preliminary steps were invisible for the doctors and their patients alike. Nevertheless, they were constitutive of the serum. The preparation of the horses and extraction of the blood fitted into a complex system with each step configuring the drug in an important way. In the next chapter, we will consider the evaluation procedure that constituted a crucial step in the requalification of the serum before it left the doors of the Pasteur Institute ready for use in a clinical setting.

NOTES

1. Johann Wolfgang von Goethe, *Faust*, Part I. Scene 4. line 214. 'Blut ist ein ganz besondrer Saft.'

2. Emil Behring and Shibasaburo Kitasato 'Ueber das Zustandekommen der Diphtherie-Immunität und der Tetanus-Immunität bei Thieren,' *Deutsche Medicinische Wochenscrift* n° 49 (1890), p. 1114.

3. For a detailed history of Behring and the early years of serum production in Germany, see Carola Throm, *Das Diphtherieserum: ein neues Therapieprinzip, seine Entwicklung und Markteinfuhrung* (Heidelberg: Wissenschaftliche Verlagsgesellschaft, 1995).

4. Erich Wernicke 'Zur Geschichte des Diphtherieserums' *Zeitschrift für ärztliche Fortbildung*, 80.5 (1931), 159–60. For more details on Wernicke's collaboration with Behring, see Erika Schulte, 'Der Anteil Erich Wernickes an der Entwicklung des Diphtherieantitoxins'(Medical thesis, Freie Universität, 2000).

5. Axel Hüntelmann, 'Diphtheria Serum and Serotherapy. Development, Production and Regulation in Fin de Siècle Germany,' *Dynamis*, 27 (2007), 107–31, on page 108.

6. 'To reconstitute natural objects as technical objects, they must be "de-worlded," artificially separated from the context in which they are originally found so as to be integrated into a technical system.' Andrew Feenberg, *Questioning Technology*, (London: Routledge, 1999), p. 203.

7. While all vertebrates have blood, the crocodile icefish (*Channichthydamodee*) have few or no red blood cells. Johan T. Ruud, 'Vertebrates without Erythrocytes and Blood Pigment' *Nature* 173, 4410 (1954): 848–850.

8. Bleeding to produce Halal meat is not, of course, to be confused with ritual animal sacrifice, another set of practices that turn around animal blood, Tahire O. Kocturk, 'Food Rules in the Koran,' *Food & Nutrition Research*, 46, 3 (2002), p. 139.

9. The toxin was first isolated by Emile Roux and Alexandre Yersin in 1888 as part of a range of experiments they carried out involving the diphtheria bacillus. Emile Roux and Alexandre Yersin 'Contribution à l'étude de la diphthérie,' *Annales de l'Institut Pasteur* 2.12 (1888) 629–61.

10. It is difficult to overestimate the contribution of animal models in human disease at this time. Without the identification of animals susceptible to diphtheria like the guinea pig and the horse, the production of the serum would have been impossible.

11. Louis Martin, 'Production de la toxine diphtérique.' (Paris: Faculté de Médecine, 1897), p. 22.

12. Louis Pasteur was the founder of one of the leading schools in early microbiology along with Robert Koch in Berlin. Every year the Pasteur Institute offered a course in 'microbie' where the first generations of French microbiologists learned their trade and a large number of medical doctors discovered this new field. For more about this course, see Chapter 6.

13. Georges Lemière, *La Diphtérie et son traitement par la sérumthérapie*, (Lille: L. Danel, 1895) p. 33.

14. Emile Roux 'Discours de M. le Dr Roux, Directeur de l'Institut Pasteur.' in *Edmond Nocard 1850–1903, Discours prononcés à la cérémonie d'inauguration du monument élevé à sa mémoire*. (Paris, Masson & Cie, n.d.), p. 46.

15. Some animals were also kept at the Veterinary School in Maisons Alfort, where Nocard could more easily monitor their progress. As Roux suggested in his speech cited above, Nocard's service became a valuable extension of the Pasteur Institute in the initial period of production. As early as 1894, the city of Paris provided additional facilities for the horses at the 'abattoir de Grenelle' a disused slaughterhouse near the Institute, Archives Municipales de Paris, DX6 8.

16. A former cavalry installation, 'les cent gardes,' was a sizable estate that had been made available to Pasteur by the government free of charge for his rabies research in 1884.

17. Aristotle *The Physics*, 199a.

18. For more on the handling of the horses, see Jonathan Simon. 'Monitoring the Stable at the Pasteur Institute' *Science in Context* 21, n° 2 (2008): pp. 181–200.

19. As we shall see later, many provincial centers set up their own serum production facilities, but none competed with the Pasteur Institute at the national level.

20. Anon. 'Le vaccin du croup' *Le Matin*, vendredi 12 octobre 1894, p. 2. A l'Institut Pasteur, on se bornera à aménager, au premier étage du pavillon réservé jusqu'à ce jour aux cages des lapins, un grand laboratoire spécialement organisé pour la préparation et l'expédition du vaccin. Deux médecins seront préposés, sous la direction permanente de M: Roux, a cette préparation du sérum, qui nécessite tant de précautions et tant de soins.

21. The testing of the quality of the serum discussed in the next chapter was also performed at Garches. Seen as a scientific step in the production process, it was

entrusted to male laboratory workers posted to Marnes-la-Coquette rather than to the female production staff hired in Paris.

22. For a discussion of the structuring and functioning of modern office work in a similar period, see Delphine Gardey, *La dactylographe et l'expéditionnaire: histoire des employés de bureau : 1890–1930* (Paris: Belin, 2001).

Chapter 3

Transforming Serum into a Medical Drug

A key step in the making of a technological object is the redefinition of the constitutive material in terms of its intended use. This is a complement to the stripping of properties discussed in the previous chapter, we can think of it as the first step in a re-worlding process, although Feenberg reserves this latter term for the elements he presented under the heading of secondary instrumentalization. In the 'ideal' configuration the overall analysis of a technological object—in this case a medical drug—would describe its transfer or, to borrow a term now only too familiar in science studies, its translation from the natural to a technological world. This translation is not a simple passage of a predefined object from one context to another, it has to be reconstituted and inserted as a technological object into a system. The object has a sense and existence within this system, but the system is not pre-established, ready to receive the object. At one and the same time, the object configures the overall structure and is in turn reconfigured by its use in this particular context.

As a first approach then, we can think about the properties or qualities of the constitutive material, those characteristics associated with the function of the object in its natural context. We see them stripped away and new ones defined in their place. This approach has the advantage of allowing us to deploy the classic philosophical opposition between the natural and the artificial.

Nevertheless, in the case of therapeutic serum, it is problematic to consider the blood circulating in the horses from which the serum was derived as a natural product, because the immunization process used to prepare the horses prior to the bleeding involved an artificial transformation of the animal. Still, whether natural or not, the question remains of how the product removed from the horse becomes a medical drug. To answer this question we need to think about what exactly constitutes a medical drug as a distinct category, and the transformations that were necessary for the serum to attain this status. In the previous chapter we presented the selection and immunization of the horses and the steps involved in transferring 10 or 20 cubic centimeters of the blood serum from these animals into a glass phial at the Pasteur Institute. In this chapter we will follow a more conceptual transformation, albeit one grounded in very real, material processes.

The transformation of this physical phial into a medical drug can be analyzed, at least in an initial approach, using Feenberg's idea of reduction. In this process, as Feenberg conceives it, the qualities of the material are redefined, bringing to the fore those that will be mobilized in its new function. Thus, the material in its new artificial form is reduced to the features that make it useful as a technological object. The questions we need to answer here, then, are, what are the relevant features in this case and how is this reduction carried out in practice? This brings us back to the central question; how does the serum become a medical drug? In this chapter we will consider this question from the perspective of the evaluation process and the serum's legal status.

The technological object as it is deployed in human society possesses certain properties or qualities[1] that were not present or at least not 'usable' in the original material at the moment it was extracted from its natural environment, and are related to the object's function in its new technological incarnation. Framed in these terms, it is hard to avoid the question of the pre-existent or persistent nature of these properties, a question we will consider in more depth later in this chapter. Putting this issue to one side for the moment, however, we can note that the central definitive property for the serum once it becomes a medical drug is its specific therapeutic efficacy, its putative capacity to cure the disease of diphtheria in human subjects. The 'objective' question, which has often been posed in the literature, as to whether this capacity was real and effective is not our principal concern here. In other words, I do not aim to answer the question that so many people have asked; did the anti-diphtheria serum cure diphtheria? Instead, I want to explore the mechanisms by which this therapeutic property was established for the anti-diphtheria serum to the satisfaction of the majority, if not all of those touched by the disease and this treatment. This investigation will cover, among other things, the concrete activities performed within the centers for production that brought the serum to the threshold of the doctor's clinic.

It is tempting to consider that the serum was already present as an active medical drug in the blood of the horses immunized against diphtheria. After all, one could argue that the effectiveness of the serum against the disease was established thanks to the prior immunization of the horses, a procedure laid out in the previous chapter. The blood serum of a horse that had never been immunized against diphtheria would be ineffective against the disease while the blood serum of an immunized animal would have therapeutic value. Following the immunization of the horse, the work seems to have been done; the serum of the immunized animal is already a medical drug. This interpretation seems to be supported by an unusual story reported in a medical journal from Montpellier (the *Montpellier médical*) in 1894. It concerns a certain doctor Bonafoux who, the article explains, lost his life in the line of duty (*mort au champ d'honneur*). The doctor accidentally contracted diphtheria due to the projection of infected material during a tracheotomy he was performing on a patient, a relatively rare but not unheard-of event. As no serum was available to treat him, the doctor was injected with blood taken from a young girl in the same Montpellier hospital who was recovering from diphtheria and so 'in a state of immunization.'[2] But this kind of experimental use of blood as a treatment, even if it is based on the principle of serotherapy, is quite exceptional, underlining the opposition with the administration of commercial serum, which was rapidly becoming the accepted norm for the treatment of diphtheria. To see this difference clearly, it is important to understand the passage of the serum to its position as a recognized medical drug. This implies two related transformations: first, removing the serum from local experimental practices to place it in the ranks of the accepted medicines of the day. Second, the operations required to turn the phial filled with serum with which we ended the last chapter into an officially sanctioned treatment acceptable for use by practicing doctors. Here, we will examine two aspects of this latter transformation in some detail; on one hand, the technical interventions and manipulations required to mark the passage from an undefined (both legally and commercially) liquid to a medical drug and, on the other, the administrative system in which the process was inscribed.

An examination of how the serum became qualified (practically and officially) as a medicine opens up a number of avenues for investigation, but we will limit ourselves here to a consideration of the practical work of evaluating the immunizing power of the serum and the integration of this innovative product into the legal structures that governed medical drugs in France at the end of the nineteenth century. Although one could make the argument that the use of statistics concerning the clinical efficacy of the serum also contributed to the definition of its properties, I will reserve my treatment of this issue for Chapter 4.

EVALUATING THE IMMUNIZING POWER: RITES OF PASSAGE

After being separated from the red blood cells, the serum was tested using guinea pigs and assigned a number that was intended to convey the potency of the product in its use against diphtheria. This testing, which we will describe in more detail below, was considered essential in a context where the immunizing power of any single batch of serum could vary not only between different horses but even between consecutive bleedings from the same horse. This variability was attributed to the fluctuations in a horse's level of immunity, which regular injections of toxin aimed to keep as high as possible. Serum producers soon realized, however, that the results of this system for managing a horse's immunity to diphtheria toxin were not entirely predictable. In these circumstances, the evaluation of immunization power performed on each and every batch of serum was introduced right from the beginning as the minimum guarantee of the effectiveness of the product and was, it appears, always performed prior to the distribution of phials of serum for use by physicians. This guarantee of efficacy was considered to be particularly important for a treatment against diphtheria, a disease that needed to be treated as early as possible in order to maximize the chances of success. Indeed, treatment with an ineffective serum was seen to pose a dual threat. First, the treating physician exposed the patient to the risks associated with the injection—at the very least cutaneous reaction and a very real possibility of serious infection—with no expected benefit. This risk was aggravated by the fact that the majority of diphtheria patients receiving this treatment would be children. At the same time, by using an ineffective product, the doctor was delaying the administration of an effective one. If there was one thing that the partisans of the serum agreed upon, it was that the earlier the treatment could be administered the better the patient's prognosis, and that delaying the treatment too long greatly increased the risk of death from the disease. In his book on serotherapy from 1898, Louis Landouzy justified this approach in terms of the nature of diphtheria, more specifically the fact that the bacteria produced a deadly toxin.

> Diphtheria is much more an intoxication than an infection, and all those who have treated it with antitoxic serum have declared that if the intervention is late, if the injection is made at a moment when the intoxication has had the time to graft itself onto the local infection, the treatment risks being ineffective.[3]

Whatever the precise explanation that might be offered—and opinions differed as we shall see in the next chapter—clinical wisdom concurred with the results of theoretical speculation in advising the administration of an effective serum at the earliest possible opportunity. Hence the importance of assigning a figure to the phials of serum indicating their immunizing power as a guarantee that such a treatment was actually being administered. But this practice quickly became more than just a guarantee that the doctor would be administering an authentic anti-diphtheria serum. Indeed, the evaluation of the immunizing power of therapeutic serum is of capital importance in the history of pharmaceutical medicine on several levels. First, because it served as a model for the codification of bioassays of drugs whether they were of biological origin or not. Thus, the immunization unit for these antitoxins became the reference for a new set of standards that would be an important element in refounding modern medicine on scientific grounds. The standardization of sera even became a model for international cooperation around medical standards, with the League of Nations Health Organization deciding at its very first meeting in 1921 to focus on sera and serological tests.[4] The fact that an organization like the League of Nations could even consider establishing an international standard is itself evidence of the status that the evaluation of the immunizing power of serum had achieved in the early twentieth century. Indeed, thanks in large part to the pioneering work of Paul Ehrlich at the turn of the century, the antitoxic action of blood sera had become one of the most highly sophisticated areas of theoretical and experimental medical research.[5] Furthermore, this work on sera was at the heart of Ehrlich's receptor theory that would prove so influential in twentieth-century pharmacology and the life sciences more generally.[6] Nevertheless, Ehrlich's elaboration of the mechanism of action of antitoxins (and later other medicines) had quite modest beginnings, originating in the observations of the variability of the effectiveness of supposedly equivalent antitoxins against diphtheria toxin.

Starting in 1891, so even before the commercialization of the serum in Germany, Ehrlich was given the task of overseeing the evaluation of its immunizing power. In Berlin and later in Frankfurt, he undertook extensive experiments to determine with precision the power of different sera to neutralize toxins. Ehrlich distinguished himself among the scientists working on these questions by his desire to have an exact mathematical description of the action of the serum against toxins, setting his goals very high, notably in terms of precision.

> It is beyond question that, in dealing with the problem of the diphtheria curative serum, whether from the practical therapeutic, or the purely scientific point of view, it is necessary to use sera of *precisely known value*.[7]

Multiplying carefully calibrated experiments, Ehrlich was forced to abandon his initial hypothesis that a unit of serum (determined in terms of immunizing power) would neutralize a certain quantity of toxin, as the experimental predictions did not fit with the results. In a series of tests, he neutralized various toxins using the same unit of antitoxin (relying on desiccated vacuum packed samples produced by Hoechst under Behring's supervision), and then determined the difference in the quantity of toxin required to kill a 250 gram guinea pig (Ehrlich always regarded this lethal dose as the most stable point in a world of fluctuating biological 'standards,' and the 250-gram guinea pig came to impose itself as the German standard). This marginal toxicity of the different toxins, which, according to Ehrlich's original model should have been proportional to the volume neutralized by the unit of antitoxin, varied by a factor of almost thirty. Such fluctuation translated into an unacceptably large margin for error, forcing Ehrlich to rethink the mechanism of the neutralization of toxin by the serum. His solution to this enigma and the general problem of the variability in toxin strength was to postulate the existence of three additional forms of toxin, which were no longer toxic and that he collectively referred to as toxoids. The three toxoids—protoxoids, syntoxoids and epitoxoids—were distinguished by their affinity for the antitoxin relative to the active toxin. The varying capacity of these harmless substances to combine with the antitoxin was used to explain the differences in the amount of toxin available after neutralization, as well as the variations in the liberation or absorption of toxin following the addition of any given toxin/toxoid mixture. This complex ontology of toxins and toxoids provided not only the mathematical variables that Ehrlich needed to model his experimental results but also a way of thinking about the variability in the 'strength' of toxins. It could then serve as the theoretical support for a new method for determining the immunization power of the serum, which relied on a standard toxin and was based on a neutralization procedure. Thus a lethal dose of toxin was mixed with varying amounts of the serum to determine the level at which no reaction took place when the mixture was injected into a 250-gram guinea pig. This technique depended for its reliable functioning on the standard toxin and the complex precautions needed to take into account the possible presence of toxoids.

This delicate (and still somewhat approximate) process was, for Ehrlich, a poor substitute for the ideal that had long been established in pharmaceutical practice; simply weighing a pure substance.

> If it ever becomes possible to obtain the antitoxin or the toxin in pure form, the preparation of standard testing-solutions will be based on a simple weighing operation and it will be unnecessary to adopt any precautions for maintaining the constancy of the standard.[8]

In the absence of such pure substances, 'it seemed impossible to relate the unit of antitoxin to the number of units of a toxin neutralized by it, with the mathematical precision which is so indispensably required for the purposes of an official test (*für prüfungsamtliche Zwecke*).' Ehrlich's future career and financial prosperity would depend on just such a test, and the elaborate government oversight of production in Germany. The requirement that companies test their anti-diphtheria serum at Ehrlich's Institute in Frankfurt provided regular income used to finance other research. Nevertheless, as Anne Hardy has pointed out, these tests had a value to companies producing serum beyond the legal requirements, as firms sought testing for the tetanus serum even when no such testing was required by law.[9]

Unlike the German serum producers, however, the Pasteur Institute in France continued to use the evaluation system devised by Behring, a procedure abandoned by its inventor as early as 1893. Indeed, an examination of the surviving registers at the Pasteur Institute suggests that they were still using this form of testing in the early decades of the twentieth century, when most of their international competitors were using a version of Ehrlich's method and everyone, including the Pasteur Institute was putting the associated antitoxin units on the label of their serum.

The French system relied on the death or survival of a series of guinea pigs as the basis for their evaluation, and was relatively straightforward. The first step was to establish a value for a lethal dose of toxin. Even without the elaborate concerns raised by Ehrlich, the scientists of the Pasteur Institute were still quite aware of the variability of the diphtheria bacteria and their capacity to produce toxin. As we have seen, the question was at the core of Louis Martin's medical thesis, and although his principal concern was the laboratory production of toxin to be injected into the horses, the lesson of the variability in the strength of the toxin used to evaluate the immunizing power of the serum did not escape him. The uncertainty concerning the toxicity of each batch of culture meant that they all had to be tested. For this, the scientists established the lethal dose of the toxin, which was the minimum volume needed to kill an animal of 500 grams within twelve hours (the Pasteur Institute worked with guinea pigs between about 320 and 550 grams—a feature that Madsen pointed out as constituting an unnecessary expense when he compared the German and the French systems in 1897).[10] Once the lethal dose had been established for a batch of toxins, it could be used for the evaluation procedure, which consisted of two separate tests for each batch of serum.

These tests involved injecting two different guinea pigs with specific quantities of serum (1/50 000th and 1/100 000 of the animal's body weight) followed by the lethal dose of the toxin established in the first step. If only the first guinea pig survived this lethal dose, then the serum was assigned a value of 150 units, and if both survived, 200 units. If both guinea pigs died then the batch of serum was rejected as insufficiently active. In 1897, the Danish bacteriologist Thorvald Madsen pointed out several weaknesses in the French approach compared to the German one. Interestingly, the problems that Madsen highlighted were not so much to do with the quality of the French serum (whether it was of low or variable quality) as with the excessive time and cost of the system in place at the Pasteur Institute. Compared to an approach where one could be satisfied with the immediate reaction of the guinea pig (or, more precisely, a lack of any reaction), having to wait for the animals to die over a period of two days was evidently inefficient.

Nevertheless, while others across Europe and the United States would adopt Ehrlich's neutralization approach, Roux and his colleagues saw no need to follow suit. At some time around 1900, the Pasteur Institute in turn started to put the Ehrlich antitoxin units on their phials of serum, but they were simply converting the older units into its equivalent in the 'universal' units that had become the accepted standard. But why did the Pasteur Institute not just convert to Ehrlich's method with the economies that this would have represented? The reason for this resistance was probably to do with national pride and a desire to remain independent, as adopting the German method would have obliged the French to adopt German standards, notably the standard toxin provided by Ehrlich's Institute in Frankfurt. Furthermore, Roux had already commented on the issue as early as 1894, he considered Ehrlich's more sophisticated evaluation procedure to be more trouble than it was worth.

> To tell the truth, we don't attach a great deal of importance to all these complicated definitions and we believe that the search for this degree of precision that is not found in nature is too much [unnecessary] effort. The essential thing is to understand one another.[11]

It might seem surprising to a modern reader that two such different systems could exist in neighboring countries without posing a serious problem in a domain as sensitive as the manufacture of pharmaceutical products. The culture of cross-border standards is now so well established in modern society that it is difficult to accept any arguments against it. Nevertheless, Roux's criticisms of Ehrlich's 'complicated definitions' were not unjustifiable, notably in light of the variability of the clinical use of the serum. Once the serum was no longer in short supply, it was not uncommon for doctors to continue injecting 10 cc doses once or several times a day until the symptoms started to abate. Each had his own rules to guide him, but the serum was administered once or multiple times based on clinical judgment.[12] In light of this quite approximate clinical use of the serum, the most important thing was to know that the serum contained antitoxin, and even an approximate idea of its relative potency would be sufficient.

Secondly, the markets in France and Germany were almost completely independent, initially de facto, and later by the force of law. We will examine the terms of the law of April 1895 that covered the serum in France and the effect that this law had in terms of structuring the French market for serum in what follows. Beyond the influence of this law, however, the economic and administrative (as well as ideological) construction of the French serum economy around the Pasteur Institute made it a market apart. The cheap and often free French serum massively dominated the domestic market and left little room for more expensive foreign products. This configuration meant that the French serum did not share the competitive context of Germany, where more sophisticated evaluation methods could give one company the edge over its competitors in the struggle for market share. To all intents and purposes, the only serum available in France was that produced by the Pasteur Institute. We will explore the paradoxical existence of local serum producers in Chapter 8, but first we will look at what precisely the law required of serum, notably in terms of the evaluation of its efficacy.

THE LEGAL STATUS OF THE SERUM

The evaluation procedure described above allowed the producers, like the Pasteur Institute, to indicate the immunization power of the serum on a label glued onto the phial. This number and the other information printed on the label were important elements in the transformation of serum into a medical drug. Although it rarely attracts much attention in the history of pharmacy, the label is an essential element (required by law since at least the eighteenth century in certain cases) in the passage from generic substance (whether physiologically active or not) to medicine. Looking closely at the label on a phial of French serum from 1910 (Figure 3.1), we can read the following:

INSTITUT PASTEUR de PARIS, FRANCE
SERVICE DE SÉROTHÉRAPIE, 22, rue Dutot
SÉRUM ANTIDIPHTÉRIQUE
Dix Centimètres Cubes
Unités antitoxiques 2.500
Pouvoir antimicrobien 1/100 000e

In a concise manner, the label informs us of the nature of the phial's contents while quantifying its essential characteristics. It is significant that the name of the producer, the Pasteur Institute, precedes the name of the product 'anti-diphtheria serum' as at this time French legislation placed more emphasis on the manufacturer of the product than the nature of the product itself. This official label is an important step, therefore, in establishing the product as a particular medical drug. The phial is not the same object with or without its label; in an important sense it becomes anti-diphtheria serum only thanks to this piece of paper. By 1896, the Pasteur Institute was already producing anti-tetanus and other sera, so the mention that the contents are for the treatment of diphtheria is relatively important. French pharmacists, like others in Europe and the US were selling increasing numbers of products that they had not prepared themselves, and it would be impossible for them to distinguish between anti-tetanus and anti-diphtheria serum without the label. The antitoxic units, determined by the tests on guinea pigs outlined above, also feature on the label. By the time this phial was produced, the French had ceded to

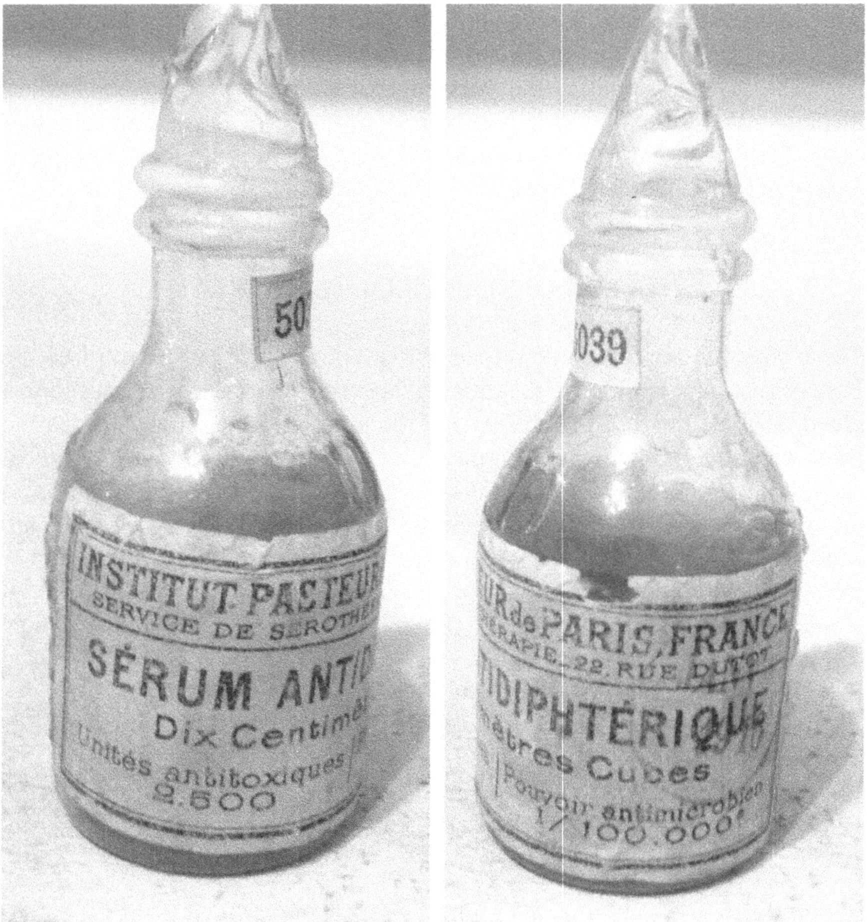

Figure 3.1 A 10 cc phial of anti-diphtheria serum produced by the Pasteur Institute, from 1910. Photograph by the author.

the pressure to adopt the international standard of antitoxin units, although, as we explained above, this did not mean they had adopted Ehrlich's testing process, and the label features an additional indication of 'antimicrobial power.' The volume of the serum is also indicated on the label, although after over a decade of widespread use of this product this would have been a relatively unimportant element of information for any experienced physician.[13]

THE PROPERTIES OF DRUGS IN A LEGAL CONTEXT

As I presented the evaluation process, I suggested on several occasions that the Pasteur Institute had certain responsibilities regarding the product. The label, for example, is informational in at least two senses; and this for any medical drug, even today. It provides the consumer (meant literally in this case) with information and the product itself. When commenting on the label on the phial, I suggested that its layout conformed to certain legal requirements. Indeed, when you read the informational inserts that accompany every packaged prescription drug today, it is clear that their layout (in particular the sections identified by clear subheadings; posology, side-effects, etc.) is largely determined by precise requirements—usually imposed by central authorities—and there is not a great deal of room for originality. The development of this labeling is a history of a constant interplay between informal standards and legal requirements, but to write a history of drug labeling would require another book. In 1894, the Pasteur Institute was quite unconstrained by the law, but starting in 1895 this was no longer the case. This, being said, at no point in the history of serum manufacture did the law dictate how the serum should be presented. What were, then, the legal requirements and restrictions placed on the serum manufacturers? The short answer is that in France, until April 1895, there were none at all. The long answer is quite complex, but it will help us to understand the full significance of this label and the manner in which the serum was qualified as a medical drug. Indeed, April 1895 constitutes a watershed in this history, as it was the moment when a text was signed into law that cleared up a situation that had been until then rather foggy, to say the least. To better understand the impact of this law, it will help to trace the first years of the serum's use in France and the evolution of the legislation that accompanied the adoption of this new product across the country.

In the presentation they made in Budapest Roux, Chaillou and Martin claimed that they started using the serum at the *Hôpital des Enfants-Malades* in February 1894, but the records of the Assistance Publique in Paris indicate its first use on January 30, 1894.[14] On that day the three men went to the diphtheria ward and 'practiced a new style of treatment on the wards.'[15] Neither these three members of the Pasteur Institute nor the hospital sought to obtain any kind of consent from the patients or their families, as all they needed for this kind of experimental treatment was the permission of the director of the diphtheria ward, Dr. Jules Simon. This clinical test of the new product was quite possibly illegal, but not, as anyone familiar with modern ethical rules for clinical trials might imagine, because of the way it was conducted. The 'chef de service' had complete power over his ward, and his permission was sufficient for any kind of experiment that lay within the limits of French criminal and civil laws.[16]

The reason that this practice may have been illegal concerns the status of the serum itself at the beginning of 1894; Was it a medical drug or not? If it was a medical drug, then its use at the hospital without the collaboration of a pharmacist was, strictly speaking, illegal. The description given at the *Hôpital des Enfants-Malades* is interesting in this respect, as it remains uncommitted as to what serotherapy was, describing it simply as 'un nouveau mode de traitement'—a new type of treatment. While today the frontier between medical drug (in French, a *médicament*) and non medical drug is in principle clearly defined by the law, this was not the case in 1894.[17] Pharmacy at that time was governed by a law dating from 1803, which provided only an implicit definition of a medical drug. Thus, while article 25 of the so-called law of Germinal (April 1803, or Germinal year XI) explicitly granted the monopoly over all medical drugs to the pharmacist, the law did not define what counted as a medical drug.[18] This law of Germinal, prepared after the French revolution was conceived for a conservative pharmaceutical culture, where the security of the supply of medical drugs did not take into account the possibility or the need for innovation in the pharmacopoeia. While the circular definition of a medical drug as the object of the pharmacist's monopoly could work satisfactorily in a context where there were few if any new drugs, it was ill adapted to a régime of innovation. By the end of the nineteenth century many new products that one would intuitively class as medical drugs were being proposed to the public, and producers flooded into the legal gray area that such innovation opened up.[19] One way of breaking out of the circular definition based on the monopoly of the pharmacists was to refer to the national pharmacopoeia, which was meant to list all the standard medical drug. The editions of this official Codex appeared so infrequently, however, that the demand for any new treatment (and so also its supply) was established well before it could be inscribed in this publication. Thus, therapeutic sera only started to appear in the French pharmacopoeia well into the twentieth century.

In the absence of any legal definition of a medical drug, therefore, the serum, like the rabies treatment that had allowed Pasteur to raise money for his Institute in the first place, slipped between the cracks in the legislation. Had the serum been officially determined to be a medical drug (in a court decision, for example) then it could, in the terms of the 1803 law, only be produced and distributed (even free of charge) by a qualified pharmacist. This would have been a serious problem for Roux (as it would have been a problem for Pasteur before him with respect to the rabies vaccine) as there was not a single qualified pharmacist on the staff of the Pasteur Institute during this period. The absence of a pharmacist meant that the Institute had no legal right to produce or distribute a medical drug. Nevertheless, Roux went ahead with production on the model of the rabies vaccine, benefiting from the unclear status of the product and operating within the loose limits of the legislator's tolerance.[20]

But diphtheria was not rabies, and French serotherapy could not be confined to the Pasteur Institute. When in January 1895, the serum started to be distributed on a national scale, the government intervened. On January 14, 1895, the Ministry of the Interior sent out a circular to all the prefects in the country.

> Monsieur le préfet, The Pasteur Institute is now able to respond to the demands for antidiphtheria serum addressed to it. The sick capable of paying for the medical drug can obtain it from pharmacists; it will be provided free of charge to the indigent.[21]

While this circular did not provide the serum with any specific legal status, the fact that the Ministry of the Interior was taking responsibility for organizing its distribution made it de facto legitimate, apparently official and by extension probably legal. Furthermore, the fact that it was to be sold by pharmacists meant that it was in all probability a medical drug. Thus, the serum entered a new phase of its legal limbo. We will return in more detail to this period of uncertainty when we look in more detail at the legislation around the serum in the penultimate chapter. To cut a long story short, the legal situation was finally resolved a year after the first use of the anti-diphtheria serum, thanks to legislation hurriedly pushed through the French National Assembly specifically aimed at sera and a range of related products. Thus, starting from April 1895, serum sold (or given away) in France had to be manufactured by an officially approved producer. The Pasteur Institute was at the top of the first list of approved producers published by the Ministry of the Interior, and so, starting from the end of 1895, the name on the label assumed a particular legal significance.[22]

The approval process was conducted by a team of experts nominated by a committee of the Ministry of the Interior. On its visits to the facilities, the team paid particular attention to the evaluation procedure for the serum, although without imposing any particular norms for how to establish the immunizing power of the drug. In light of the rapid approval given to the Pasteur Institute for its anti-diphtheria serum, we have to assume that their technique fully satisfied the standards of the time, at least in France. Once tested and labeled, the serum could be sent out for use.

Following the very early period of production when doctors had knocked at the door of the Pasteur Institute to receive the serum directly from Roux or one of his colleagues, the dispatch room became the last point of contact between the producers and the serum. The dispatchers carefully packaged the phials of serum and noted in ledgers where the different packages were being sent. Apparently as early as 1895, the serum could be ordered by means of a telegraph message addressed to 'SERPASTEUR-PARIS.'

Unlike the Germans, the French asked for nothing in return from the doctors who were going to use the serum. While Hoechst had put in place a system whereby doctors were to file reports of their use of the medicine by filling out forms packaged with the product, the French included only instructions for use. Indeed, in 1896 an initiative by Dr. Sevestre to collect this kind of information proposed to the Medical Society of the Paris Hospitals (*la Société médicale des hôpitaux de Paris*) was put to the vote and rejected.[23] The

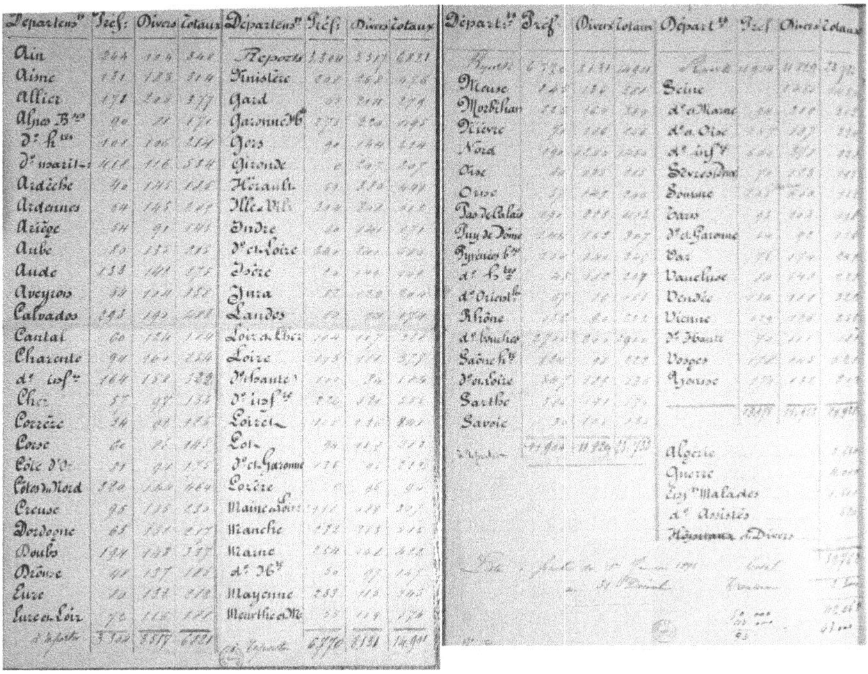

Figure 3.2 The quantities of serum distributed by the Pasteur Institute to each department in France in 1895. Photograph by the author, Institut Pasteur- Archives

principal argument put forward by members of the Society against Sevestre's 21-item questionnaire was that it would be an unacceptable constraint for the practicing physician, with professional sensibilities clearly outweighing the putative interest of such a clinical enquiry.

The product as it was sent out by the Pasteur Institute was now defined in terms of its curative qualities. Endowed with a specific legal status, what attended the serum next was its use by doctors in cases of suspected diphtheria (for the amounts of serum dispatched to the different *Départements* in 1895, see Figure 3.2). In the next chapter, we will see what arguments were mobilized to convince doctors that these products with their immunity units inscribed on the labels would translate into clinical success on the diphtheria wards of hospitals and in the homes of the patients.

NOTES

1. Feenberg uses the term primary qualities (and also, later on, the complementary term secondary qualities), although this vocabulary does not correspond with the long philosophical tradition of the use of these terms. Andrew Feenberg, *Questioning Technology*, 1999.

2. This case is reported in another journal *Lyon médical* 77, p. 488.

3. Louis Landouzy, *Les sérothérapies: leçons de thérapeutique et matière médicale*, (Paris: G. Carré et C. Naud, 1898), p. 215.

4. Pauline M. H. Mazumdar 'The State, the Serum Institutes and the League of Nations' in Simon and Gradmann (eds), *Evaluating and Standardizing Therapeutic Agents, 1890–1950*. (Basingstoke: Palgrave Macmillan, 2010), p. 119.

5. It is interesting to note that Henry Hallett Dale who worked on the standardization of the insulin unit in the 1920s had spent time in Ehrlich's Institute in Frankfurt. Christiane Sinding, 'Making the Unit of Insulin: Standards, Clinical Work and Industry, 1920–1925.' *Bulletin of the History of Medicine* 76: 2, (2002) 231–70.

6. Cay-Rüdiger Prüll 'Paul Ehrlich's Standardization of Serum: Wertbestimmung and its meaning for twentieth-century biomedicine' in Christoph Gradmann and Jonathan Simon (eds). *Evaluating and Standardizing Therapeutic Agents, 1890–1950*. (Basingstoke: Palgrave Macmillan, 2010), pp. 13–30.

7. Paul Ehrlich, 'Die Wertbemessung des Diphtherieheilserums und deren theoretische Grundlagen,' *Klinisches Jahrbuch*, 6 (1897), p. 299. English translation, Paul Ehrlich, *The collected papers of Paul Ehrlich*, F. Himmelweit et al. (eds) (London: Pergamon Press, volume 3, 1957), p.107.

8. Paul Ehrlich, 'The Assay of the Activity of Diphtheria-curative Serum and its Theoretical Basis,' in F. Himmelweit et al. (eds) *The collected papers of Paul Ehrlich*, (London: Pergamon, 1957), Vol. 3, p. 107.

9. Anne I. Hardy 'From Diphtheria to Tetanus: The Development of Evaluation Methods for Sera in Imperial Germany' in Christoph Gradmann and Jonathan Simon (eds), *Evaluating and Standardizing Therapeutic Agents, 1890–1950* (Palgrave Macmillan, 2010) pp. 52–70.

10. Thorvald Madsen, 'Ueber Messung der Stärke des antidiphtherischen Serums,' *Zeitschrift für Hygiene und Infektionskrankheiten*, 24 (1897), 437.

11. Emile Roux, and Louis Martin 'Contribution à l'étude de la diphtérie (sérum-thérapie)' (3e Mémoire) *Annales de l'Institut Pasteur, Paris* 8ème année, No. 9 (September 1894), p. 621.

12. For a more detailed examination of this clinical use of the serum based on the diphtheria ward of the *Charité* hospital in Lyon, see Jonathan Simon, 'Standardization and Clinical Use: The Introduction of the Anti-Diphtheria Serum in Lyon,' in Alexander von Schwerin et al. (eds), *Biologics: a History of Agents Made from Living Organisms in the Twentieth Century* (London: Pickering & Chatto, 2013), 33–46.

13. As we have seen, the initial unit of serum was a phial of 20 cc, but at some time around 1900, this standard unit was reduced to 10 cc. It appears that the Pasteur Institute never produced a differentiated range of volumes of serum for injection.

14. Roux, Chaillou and Martin publicly announced their results with the serum against diphtheria on the occassion of the 8th International Congress on Hygiene and Demography held in Budapest, September 1–9, 1894.

15. Archives de l'Assistance Publique—Hôpitaux de Paris, Historique des etablissements, 1894, Hôpital des Enfants-Malades, p. 289, 30 janvier 'Mr le Dr Roux et ses aides, mm. Martin et Chaillou viennent, avec l'autorisation de M. le docteur J. Simon, chargé du service de la diphtérie, pratiquer dans ces salles un nouveau mode de traitement.'

16. For a more dramatic case concerning syphilis, see Alex Dracobly, 'Ethics and Experimentation on Human Subjects in Mid-nineteenth-century France: The Story of the 1859 Syphilis Experiments,' *Bulletin of the History of Medicine*, 77, 2 (2003), 332–66.

17. A medical drug (*médicament*) is defined in French law by article L.5111–1 of the 'Code de la Santé Publique.' The definition is quite broad and depends on how the product is presented, although the definition is based on the product's (purported) physiological properties (Toute substance ou composition présentée comme possédant des propriétés curatives ou préventives à l'égard des maladies humaines ou animals.) This approach to the definition of a medical drug was only introduced in France in 1953 (Livre V, Titre 1 'Conditions générales d'exercice de la profession de pharmacien,' article 511, 1st paragraph, *Journal Officiel*, October 7, 1953, p. 8876).

18. ART. 25. Nul ne pourra obtenir de patente pour exercer la profession de pharmacien, ouvrir une officine de pharmacie, préparer, vendre ou débiter aucun médicament, s'il (n'est pas dûment qualifié comme pharmacien).

19. The term secret remedy (*remède secret*) covered any medical drug whose ingredients were unknown.

20. It is hard to believe that Louis Pasteur never reflected on this problem, as he was very careful not to infringe on the medical profession's monopoly by administering the new anti-rabies treatment himself. This caution led to his close collaboration with Dr. Jacques-Joseph Grancher, who after injecting the vaccine into Joseph Meister headed the first vaccination center in Paris.

21. F. Phily, *Jurisprudence générale et législation de la médecine-pharmacie à l'usage des médecins, chirurgiens, pharmaciens, dentistes, sages-femmes, vétérinaires, herboristes. Décisions de toutes les juridictions . . . publiées depuis quinze ans (1895–1910)* (Paris: Administration du Recueil des sommaires de la jurisprudence francaise, 1911), p. 731

22. The name was also molded into the glass of the phial as was the information that it was free (for those too poor to be able to pay for it). We will go through these requirements in more detail when we treat the law more extensively later.

23. Sevestre 'Séance du 21 février 1896' *Bulletins et mémoires de la Société médicale des hôpitaux de Paris*, (1896) 204–5.

Chapter 4

Making the Serum Work

With the serum safely sealed in its phial, we can now turn our attention to the question that is most often asked about serotherapy; did it work? Was the antitoxin an effective treatment against diphtheria? This is not just a retrospective question posed by historians, it was also a question asked by those who introduced serotherapy in Germany, France, Austria, Italy or the United States. Reading the medical press from the end of the nineteenth century, we can see that a wide consensus was quickly reached that the serum was an effective treatment for diphtheria, but here I want to take the time to consider what this might mean and how this consensus was forged.

While it is a complex issue, efficacy is central in trying to understand the serum as a technology. Philosophical reflections on the nature of technological objects take as their starting point the observation that such objects multiply the force of humans in some way. Microscopes (from those that use light to scanning-electron microscopes) augment the resolving power of human eyesight, the bicycle allows people to travel faster, a system of pulleys enables people to lift weights that they could never hope to lift otherwise. The asymmetry that such technology establishes between humans and their environment is one of the striking features of the modern world: thus, the hunter feels almost nothing as her rifle recoils, and yet the deer in the telescopic sights is killed instantly by the bullet from the gun. This asymmetry, and the idea of a multiplication of the physical (and to a lesser extent mental) capacities of humans has established itself at the heart of philosophical reflections on technology.

Technology gives humans power over or in the world beyond the physical capacities of their own body. This image of technology brings certain objects to mind before others, and for most people medical drugs would not figure in the first group. The asymmetry is most readily seen in 'mechanical' objects like the internal combustion engine or a firearm, making it unsurprising that the history and philosophy of technology have, until recently, been dominated by studies of machines in their most traditional sense. In this mode, Bruno Latour has often cited the mythical story of Archimedes and his claim to Hiero of Syracuse that with a lever and a fixed external fulcrum he could move the entire earth as emblematic of technological promise. Indeed, along with the pulley, the lever remains the archetypal machine for multiplying human force, despite the proliferation of different types of machine over time.[1] But in a well-known paper from the 1980s, Latour moved beyond this foundational example to an analysis of the multiplication of forces around Louis Pasteur's laboratory itself.[2] While Latour's goal here was to argue for the importance of the laboratory (and ultimately its ubiquity) rather than to dispute what counts as technology, he nevertheless launched a number of reflections that are quite pertinent for our analysis here. In one of his characteristically playful mixing of metaphors, Latour explains how Pasteur's farming of microbes constituted a scientific parallel to the more traditional farming practices of the communities he was targeting as an eventual market for his anthrax vaccine. The solution for Pasteur, as Latour sees it, was to turn the farm (in particular on the occasion of the public demonstration of his anthrax vaccine in Pouilly le Fort) into a laboratory. While this idea of the conversion of everywhere outside into an extension of the laboratory constitutes the core of Latour's argument, reading around it we can see the pertinence of his general thinking for the present exercise. I will not here be arguing that serotherapy turned the whole of France into a bacteriological laboratory, but will instead be exploring the transformation of the social world of medicine by the introduction of a new technology. We will wait for the following chapters to see how doctors, hospitals and patients were changed by serotherapy but now is the moment to start thinking about how technologies are made effective in the 'field' of clinical practice.

Although Latour's approach is interesting in terms of how it mixes up levers and vaccines, it is not easy to see how medical drugs multiply the user's force.[3] The asymmetry of an effective treatment against a deadly disease like diphtheria is a different kind of relationship from that conveyed by the classic examples of the lever or the automobile. In the case of a medical drug, the deployment of the object is aimed at reducing suffering or, in cases like diphtheria, the risk of the patient dying. In this sense, while it does not literally multiply the actor's force, such a drug gives a power to a human that he or she would not otherwise possess. Indeed the power of vaccination to save people from smallpox is prodigious, resonating with the stories of Archimedes and the fantastic machines he developed to defend Syracuse against the most powerful invaders. At its most extreme, we can imagine that in the case of infection with a fatal disease the person will die in the absence of the drug while following its administration he or she will live.[4] Thus, we start from the initial hypothesis that this idea of an effective treatment—in a word, efficacy—can stand in as an approximate equivalent to the mechanical multiplication of human force in classic examples of technological objects.

If we understand the multiplication of force in this context as the drug's efficacy or its capacity to save patients' lives, serotherapy was far from being an instantiation of the ideal drug we characterized above. The serum, however potent, did not cure all cases of diphtheria, and, as we shall see in more detail below, it quite possibly killed a significant number of children who would have lived had they not received this treatment. On the positive side, so to speak, the majority of those who died following their treatment with serotherapy probably died from diphtheria (or would have died from diphtheria in the absence of the serotherapy) and so would not have survived anyway. While this might appear a cynical observation from a present-day perspective, we need to recall the very high mortality rate associated with the disease, particularly in young children, and the apparent therapeutic impotence of the time.[5] As with nearly all medical drugs, today as in the past, what is now termed the ratio of benefit to risk[6] is very hard to determine, and different methods for establishing this relationship led to widely divergent assessments of the serum's clinical value (both at the time, and retrospectively). Thus, it would be illusory to try to establish the serum's efficacy against diphtheria in any absolute sense, and it is better to start from the idea that the effect of asymmetry so clearly identified by the promoters of serotherapy (a relatively small risk for a considerably increased chance of surviving a deadly disease) resides at least as much in the way the medicine was perceived at the time as in its effective action in the world.

Today, the statistical analysis of the results of clinical trials where (according to the ideal model) an active principle is tested against a placebo is widely regarded as delivering a precise numerical evaluation of the advantage offered by any given medical drug against a disease condition when compared to taking no action at all.[7] Nevertheless, the only thing we can be certain that these studies provide is the results of the statistical analyses of the trials in question. Superficially, this comment might seem to constitute a cynical rejection of the clinical trial which has become the bedrock of research and decision-making for both the modern pharmaceutical industry and the associated regulation agencies around the world. But my point here is not that nothing can be learned from such trials, rather it is that for various reasons such trials fail to deliver a precise measure of the efficacy of the drug or drugs under test.

So let's try again. While the clinical trial has become the standard to which clinical practice refers (the 'gold-standard' in medicine, as other researchers have already observed), we might still be better off considering the alternative hypothesis that the nearest equivalent of mechanical advantage—at the heart of the argument for the utility of a machine—is instead to be found in laboratory research into the mode of functioning of these drugs.[8] It is one of the enduring ironies of pharmaceutical research that such theory-oriented 'fundamental' research is notoriously difficult to translate into clinical outcomes (hence the reliance on a range of empirical practices such as drug screening for drug discovery and the clinical trial for establishing efficacy—it would be inconceivable, for example, to plan a flight to Mars based on similar principles). This being said, the elucidation of fundamental mechanisms contributes a great deal to winning the hearts and minds of the clinicians who are asked to prescribe a drug to their patients and, more recently, the investors who finance the pharmaceutical industry. You need only look at a publication on an innovative cancer drug, to take this area of research as an example, to see the importance of a plausible anti-tumoral mechanism in the presentation of the molecule under trial. Thus, these often quite speculative mechanisms constitute an important element in the construction of a drug's utility, even though the regulatory arguments for its use have to be based on the results of clinical trials.[9] No government body like the FDA or the EMA[10] would consider approving a new drug in the absence of statistical arguments in its favor based on clinical trials. Nevertheless, while it is conceivable that these agencies would give their approval in the absence of any plausible mechanism for a drug's action, such a case remains highly improbable. The point of this digression is to argue for the importance of the twin criteria of clinical trials and biological mechanism that have become the standard elements of proof in modern pharmacy. These two elements are relatively recent in the history of pharmacy, dating in their modern form from after the Second World War. Nevertheless, the case we will be considering here from the end of the nineteenth century contributed to both these areas, and we can see early versions of these same considerations taking shape around the serum in a way that was almost unknown before. Indeed, considering the example of Paul Ehrlich's work on the evaluation of the serum we have already seen how far the 'empirical' question of evaluating the immunizing strength of the serum carried this gifted researcher into a sophisticated theory of drug action.

Another important element in establishing confidence in the serum, and encouraging doctors to use it is the testimonial. The first-hand clinical report of the use of the treatment by physicians replete with a description of the clinical conditions and the outcome was complemented by the author's general commentary and their perception of the value (and the risks) of the serum. For most of the history of health care in the world, it was this kind of testimonial that determined the fate of a medical drug, whether it was simply at the level of word-of-mouth assurances or, increasingly in the nineteenth century, through professional publications and paid-for advertisements. And although the influence of such testimonials is difficult to assess, it is clear that they contributed to the acceptance and widespread use of serotherapy. In this chapter, therefore, we will consider these three aspects of the diphtheria serum; its efficacy as measured by statistics, the explanations for how it functioned as a treatment for the disease, and the individual clinical reports that filled the medical journals in 1895 and served as important arguments for the medical community. Thus, retrospectively, this period can be seen as marking the beginning of a change in approaches to medical drugs, with an emerging scientific orientation sitting side by side with a quite traditional attitude to the serum. On one side we can discern the beginning of innovative approaches to the assessment of the efficacy of the serum that would transform the development and regulation of drugs in the twentieth century and on the other the weight of the more traditional thinking about evaluating such products. We will start then with the innovative side, considering the rise of statistics and mechanisms of drug action and conclude with the well-worn tradition of testimonials from the medical community.

THE CLINICAL VALUE OF THE SERUM

How is efficacy established? There are those who believe that the efficacy of a pharmaceutical treatment is something inherent in the product itself and that all the techniques that are brought to bear (laboratory studies but most importantly clinical trials) are simply the means to reveal this property in an unambiguous way. As a corollary to my position on the existence of a medical drug independently of its being integrated into a system of production, approval and distribution, I would maintain that no such efficacy exists independently of the tests that are intended to bring it to light. This is not, as it may seem, a 'social constructivist' position as I would willingly admit that something exists—call it physiological activity or specific cellular action—but this does not equate to efficacy. As with the very concept of the medical drug itself, I am not searching for the correct technical definition of efficacy but will instead adopt a naturalistic approach to this idea with respect to any drug. That is to say we can understand efficacy best in terms of the means that are put into play to determine the value of this parameter. In a nutshell, we need to put the issue of the 'true' efficacy of a specific treatment against a disease to one side and see how efficacy was established in practice. An advantage of this approach is that it gives us an insight into what efficacy might mean beyond a dictionary definition. Once again, it is not that I want to question the efficacy of the serum or any other drug for that matter; it is simply that I want to examine the mechanisms that determine and evaluate this efficacy in the first place. As I have already suggested, I will be arguing that three elements established this idea that the serum was an effective treatment for diphtheria. First, there were the statistics that 'demonstrated' that serotherapy reduced mortality. Once again, I am not here concerned about whether the statistics did or did not prove what they claimed to prove, I want instead to explore how they were mobilized. The same goes for the second element, the search for a plausible mechanism of action for the serum. Here, I am not looking to see which explanation was more convincing, let alone which one was correct. Instead, I will pass in review several arguments that were made in terms of the physiology of the treated organism in order to see what kinds of argument were being made. Finally, we will turn briefly to the importance of the physician's personal experience of using the serum, with these experiences in turn often triggered by the reports published by his colleagues.

THE POWER OF NUMBERS: STATISTICAL PROOFS

One of the reasons that serotherapy has attracted the interest of modern researchers is because of the statistical arguments that were used to demonstrate its effectiveness as a specific treatment against diphtheria.[11] Starting with a particular example, albeit a very significant one for the history of serum in France, it is hard to deny that the presentation of the serum by Emile Roux in Budapest in September 1894 derived much of its impact from the impressive figures drawn from the different diphtheria wards around Paris.

Between February 1 and July 24, 1894, when the serum was being used on Dr. Simon's diphtheria ward of the *Hôpital des Enfants-Malades* in Paris, 448 children were admitted with the disease, of whom 109 died, translating into a mortality rate of 24.33%. Between 1890 and 1894 this mortality rate was on average 51.71% for a total of 3971 children on the ward; thus, all other things being equal, the benefit provided by the treatment was 27.38%. During this same period of time, 500 children entered the *Hôpital Trousseau* with diphtheria and 316 died, giving a mortality rate of 63.20%.[12]

Roux presented these numerical results of the first use of serum in France because he took them to be both proof and a measure of the efficacy of the serum against diphtheria. Indeed, a reduction of almost 30 percent in the mortality due to an infectious disease is very impressive, and the comparison with the *Hôpital Trousseau* suggests that the 'real' impact might have been even greater. The figures that were presented in Budapest did have a considerable effect, and were widely disseminated by medical journals across Europe. Others would return to the statistics regularly, as well as adding to them in one sense or another, usually with the aim of demonstrating the efficacy of the serum. Researchers, increasingly specialists in the statistics concerning

Table 4.1 Deaths from diphtheria in the 100 largest cities in France in the periods 1888–1894 and 1895.

	Deaths from diphtheria in the 100 largest cities in France		*Decrease*	
Month	*Avg 1888–1894*	*1895*	*In numbers*	*Percent*
January	469	205	264	56.2
February	466	187	279	59.5
March	499	155	344	69.3
April	442	160	282	63.8
May	417	113	304	72.5
June	333	84	249	74.5

public health, went to great lengths to estimate how many lives had been saved by this new therapy.

In his 1898 publication on serotherapy, Louis Landouzy published statistics from around the world, each more dramatic than the last. Thus, limiting ourselves to the figures from Europe, he cites a mortality rate of 22.8% from Vienna, 21% from Berlin, and in Madrid a spectacular drop from over 80% to a little under 8% following the introduction of serotherapy. While not quite as dramatic, perhaps the most surprising statistic for those acquainted with the history of public health in Europe during this period, is a reported drop in mortality rate from 50% to 12.5% in an English hospital.[13]

Landouzy goes on to present the table reproduced here, in which he compared deaths in cities in France for the same months of the year; in one column the averages for the decade between 1884 and 1894 (before the introduction of the serum) and in the other column the deaths in 1895 (Table 4.1). Based on these figures, Landouzy estimated that 15 000 lives were being saved every year across France by this treatment.

Unsurprisingly in light of his orientation in favor of the treatment, Landouzy concludes by announcing his unconditional support for serotherapy.

> Sirs, I believe I have recounted enough to prove that the hopes founded on the antidiphtheritic serum have been fully justified and that the promises made by Behring and Roux were not above the level of reality. The serotherapy for diphtheria draws its solid basis not from a few cases but from tens of thousands gathered together from the four corners of the globe.[14]

We could easily multiply the illustrations of this kind of statistical compilation published in medical journals all across the industrialized world following the introduction of the serum. For our purposes here it is enough to note the nature of this argument and how widespread it was. Taking a closer look at the various contemporary positions and the uses of statistics made by the different researchers raises a number of interesting questions.

THE PROBLEM WITH PUBLIC HEALTH STATISTICS

In a medical thesis defended at the Paris faculty of medicine in 1900, Victor Chary, with the help of the experienced public health statistician Jacques Bertillon, gathered together statistics on diphtheria from several European countries for the nineteenth century.[15] Like Landouzy, Chary's aim was to use this information to try and prove the efficacy of the serotherapy as a treatment against diphtheria, showing how the widespread introduction of this innovative therapy coincided with a significant drop in mortality from the disease. One of the striking elements in this compilation of statistics is the difference in the figures for diphtheria between France and England. Consider the situation in London and Paris for the year 1881, for example.[16] With a population of just over 3.8 million, London was a much larger city than Paris which had around 2.3 million inhabitants. By contrast, with over two thousand deaths from diphtheria, the French capital was much harder hit than its British counterpart for which Chary calculated 657 deaths due to diphtheria in 1881. He concluded that while Paris had a mortality rate of 9.9 per ten thousand inhabitants from diphtheria, London's rate, at around 1.7 per ten thousand, was over 5 times lower. Thus, it seems that England was relatively protected from the disease. Nevertheless, the next decade saw the rate of diphtheria deaths increase in London (and Britain more generally) to attain the same levels as those seen in Paris.

According to Chary's statistics, there was a lasting inversion of the situations in France and Britain that took place in the time-period around the introduction of the serotherapy. While, starting in 1895, the mortality rate from diphtheria for Paris was cut in half and remained at a consistently low level thereafter, in London it dropped only slightly, before rising again in 1896 and remaining high (Table 4.2). Thus, with the arrival of a treatment that was widely regarded as being highly effective (the French, Norwegians and

Table 4.2 Deaths from diphtheria per 10 000 inhabitants in France and in Britain.

Year	*France*	*England and Wales*	*Paris*	*London*
1891	5.19	2.6	5.6	4.2
1892	4.88	3	5.7	5.1
1893	5.98	3.9	5.2	8.1
1894	3.83	3.5	4.1	6.6
1895	1.73	3.1	1.7	5.7
1896	1.71	3.5	1.8	6.3
1897	1.22	2.9	1.2	5.3
1898	No data	2.8	1	4.1
1899	1.2	No data	1.3	4.5

Deaths per 10 000 compiled from Victor Chary, 'La mortalité par diphtérie. . .' 1900.

German specialists were certainly convinced by their own statistics) the English failed to observe the same drop in overall mortality rate from the disease.

In 1900, Louis Cobbett, a doctor from the pathological laboratory in Cambridge published a more detailed treatment of the situation in Britain city by city. While he calculated a significant drop in mortality rates (particularly when correlated with reports of the disease), there were some cities where the mortality rate was on the rise. This was the case with Liverpool, for example, where there had been an average rate of 14.8 deaths per 100,000 before the introduction of the serum and this had risen to 24.1 for the years starting in 1895.[17]

I introduce the paradoxical situation in certain cities in Britain to draw attention to the potential problems with the statistical arguments in favor of the efficacy of serotherapy against diphtheria. These statistics (among others) have given rise to a number of reflections by twentieth-century social scientists and are at the root of a fundamental debate concerning the role of modern medicine in the dramatic changes in demography in the nineteenth century. In her book on infectious disease in nineteenth-century Britain, for example, Anne Hardy offers a mitigated assessment of the effect of the serum. While the comparison of general mortality with that observed in the hospitals of the Metropolitan Asylums Board in London suggests that the serum (at first almost exclusively administered in hospitals in England) was 'moderately effective,' Hardy nevertheless arrives at the general conclusion that 'antitoxin serum assisted a natural decline in the virulence of the disease.'[18] Indeed, her main argument concerns the predominance of different strains of the *Corynebacterium diphtheriae* bacterium (characterized by their virulence, with one much deadlier than the others) to explain the rise and fall in the mortality rates.[19] Furthermore, the mortality rates, such as those presented by Chary, were based on the number of deaths, but did not take into account the number of cases of diphtheria, meaning that even if the diphtheria strain was replaced by a less virulent one, a rise in the number of cases could also account for a rise in the overall mortality rate.

These figures and the uncertainties that surround their explanation have also fed into a significant debate that flared up in the 1960s around the work of a social scientist called Thomas McKeown. The 'McKeown' thesis, as it is known, is the claim that, at least until the twentieth century, progress in medical science contributed little to the decline in the mortality due to infectious disease and the rise in life expectancy more generally.[20] One of McKeown's arguments concerns the changing virulence of the pathogens responsible for major infectious diseases as a coincidental factor in the reduction of mortality, but what comes across most clearly from his argumentation is the insecure basis provided by the general mortality statistics available at the time for concluding specific causal hypotheses.

MORE SPECIFIC PROBLEMS

The interpretation of what these statistics from the nineteenth century really show is one issue, but this is compounded by a range of fundamental problems confronting those who want to exploit this data.

One problem, which is lost in the much higher-level argument over reduction in mortality, is an absence of statistics concerning how many people were treated with serotherapy. While the statistics reported by Roux in Budapest and similar results from Berlin hospitals were very precise concerning who was and who was not treated with the serum, the global mortality figures compiled by Chary, among others, just compared different years (notably 1894 vs. 1895) encouraging the reader to assume that any difference in mortality rate was due to treatment with serum, but without giving any information about what proportion of the diagnosed population actually received this treatment. Indeed, there are, as far as I know, no global statistics on the use of serum in France from 1895 to 1900. Nevertheless, extrapolating from what we do know about a city like Lyon, we can suppose that serotherapy had a relatively high uptake in hospitals and a much lower rate of use in private practice.[21]

We also need to consider another major factor affecting these figures, which was the identification and reporting of diphtheria. As we shall see in the next chapter, when compiling his figures Chary was obliged to combine croup and diphtheria in the British statistics. This decision reflects an ongoing debate in Britain about what to include as diphtheria in the reported figures. This debate was transformed, although not entirely resolved by the generalized introduction of the microscope for making a microbiological diagnosis of the disease based on the presence of the corynebacteria in samples from patients, generally taken from the false membrane. As 'true' diphtheria increasingly came to be identified with the presence of Loeffler's bacteria, cases that previously would have been considered diphtheria (on clinical grounds) no longer qualified, and vice versa. While we will explore this large and complex domain of diagnosis and reporting in the next chapter, we raise it here as it also had a profound influence on the statistics used to argue for the efficacy of serotherapy.

Of course, it is only too easy from a modern-day perspective to criticize these statistics, as the comparisons suffer from all the faults that randomization was intended to resolve, using chance or random selection to eliminate the selection bias to which clinicians were prone. Nevertheless, while, there was clearly a lot at stake in deploying statistics in order to prove (or, for some, disprove) that the serum was effective, these figures were probably not as important as the effect the use of serum had on medical practice and the perception that doctors formed of the drug. These points will be explored in more detail later in the book, so I now want to turn to the second part of this analysis which concerns the movement to establish a plausible, if not consensual, mechanism for the action of the serum as a treatment against diphtheria.

MECHANISMS—HOW DOES THE SERUM 'REALLY' WORK?

A feature that set serotherapy apart from other drugs of the time is the integration of scientific research into both its development and its production. As we have seen, the serum's manufacture and testing involved in vitro as well as in vivo techniques, and we should recall that the origins of serotherapy was in a more or less systematic research program based on a chemical vision of anti-bacterial drug action.[22] While vaccination and its ancestors, like variolation, were based on empirically determined and developed practices, the pioneers of serotherapy were never content to rest at this level. For Behring, Roux, Ehrlich and their colleagues, the question of the serum's mechanism of action was of capital importance. In this context, the production and testing of the serum also taught these researchers a number of important lessons about the functioning if not necessarily the nature of immunity. We have already presented Ehrlich's mathematically sophisticated theory of toxins and toxoids when we dealt with the evaluation of serum, and it is worth recalling that neither this approach nor the much more influential side-chain and receptor theories would have developed in the same way without the pressing practical concerns associated with the production and evaluation of serum.

Thus, the introduction of serotherapy contributed significantly to the rise of scientific studies (notably laboratory studies) of immunity and has played an important if generally underrated role in the rise of immunology in the twentieth century. Histories of immunology are much more concerned with the foundational debate that ran through this period between proponents of a humoral theory of immunity and those who defended a cellular alternative.[23] As the focus of these histories is the development of theories of immunity they dedicate relatively little place to questions touching either the production of serum or its clinical use. A brief review of this Franco-German theoretical clash will help to illustrate the significance of laboratory work in this area.

Faithful to Robert Koch, Emil Behring favored the humoral theory in connection with the research that led him to serotherapy in 1890. As I have explained elsewhere, for Behring—at least in the beginning of his research—blood was just one item on a long list of organic chemicals that were being screened for their bactericidal properties. Nevertheless, he soon moved on from a straightforward bactericidal effect to a mechanism of neutralization. Thus, he considered that the blood serum was somehow neutralizing the toxins and thereby rendering the disease inoffensive. Neutralization was the principle behind later testing of the serum, as a pre-mixture of toxin with antitoxin in the correct quantities injected into an animal evinced no physiological reaction. Most of the researchers associated with the Koch institute not only favored this approach, which was understood to fit with the humoral tradition, but also had a chemical vision of this process. The antitoxin was considered to be a chemical match for the toxin (a version of the famous lock-and-key model developed by Emil Fischer to explain the specificity of the functioning of enzymes)[24] which, by binding to it could neutralize if not destroy it.

Paul Ehrlich supported this picture of chemical combination, but had doubts about whether the binding of the toxin to the antitoxin eliminated the toxin. Indeed, reports of experiments where 'neutralized' toxin was rendered toxic again suggested that this was not correct.

> Essentially the question to be answered is, whether neutral toxin-antitoxin mixtures (i.e., such as have become innocuous to test animals) can once more, under given conditions, develop toxic properties, a result which would be impossible if the toxin had been destroyed.[25]

Trying to weigh up the different observations, Ehrlich finally took refuge in agnosticism concerning the precise mechanism of action of the serum.

> It would be rash to draw any conclusions of a general character from the uncertain, incomplete and confused observations that exist.[26]

Despite a clear preference for a humoral, and in particular a chemical theory of the action of serum, the Germans did not manage to arrive at a very precise explanation. Thus, beyond the general sentiment that the serum acted through some kind of chemical-like (but reversible) neutralization process, there was little consensus. This being said, no researchers claimed that the serum did not in fact work, and there was widespread confidence that the correct mechanism would be identified.

In France, and at the Pasteur Institute in particular, researchers had taken a different path, reflecting, although not directly, a general preference for the biological over the chemical.[27] The most influential figure in debates around an organism's defense mechanisms against disease was the Russian-born biologist Elie Metchnikoff. Examining various marine animals under the microscope, Metchnikoff was the first to describe phagocytosis, a process where cells absorb and destroy foreign matter, particularly bacteria. Such cells, called phagocytes, could be found among the white blood cells in human blood, and he postulated this mechanism as the basis of immunity. Metchnikoff would receive a Nobel Prize for this work in 1908.[28] Those working on serum at the Pasteur Institute loyally put phagocytosis to the fore in their search for probable mechanisms, promoting the work of Metchnikoff and his disciples in this area. In an article on the diphtheria serum from 1894, Emile Roux and Louis Martin cited Georg Gabritschevsky, who was working in Metchnikoff's laboratory.

> Without wanting to deal with the important question of doctrine [phagocytosis versus humoral theory], we would say that the antidiphtheria serum is not antitoxic in the literal sense of the word; added to toxin it leaves it intact; injected into animals, it acts on their cells, rendering them, for a certain time, insensible to the poison. . . .
>
> Is not the natural explanation for these facts the action of the serum on the cells? The lively cells of new Guinea pigs respond to the stimulation of the serum; while other animals—apparently just as vigorous—which have already been marked by contact with microbial products remain defenceless when they encounter the toxin. The study of the phagocytic reaction in diphtheria has been undertaken at the Pasteur Institut by M. Gabritschevsky. The conclusions he has arrived at concur with the idea that preventive serums are stimulant and not antitoxic.[29]

This grand face-off between cellular and humoral mechanism that has been taken to open the modern science of immunology was markedly national in character, with the German community lining up behind the humoral approach, and the French adhering in the vast majority to the cellular theory.

In 1895, the Belgian specialist physician M. Funck published a comprehensive review of diphtheria serotherapy. After presenting the development of the neutralization hypotheses defended in Berlin, Funck turns to what he terms 'the Paris school' and their position that the serum is an '*excitant cellulaire*'—that it stimulates the defensive action of the cells. He concludes with an indecisive but even-handed summary.

> It is probable that we will show that a part of the truth lies with each of the two theories; the direct neutralization of the poison by its antitoxin and the exclusive action of the white cells.[30]

Landouzy's serotherapy manual published three years later paints a very similar picture, although he is, maybe for patriotic reasons, more inclined to favor the stimulant position.

> According to some authors, serotherapy—the introduction of serum into the organism—plays the role of an excitor, a dynamogen. It increases the blood pressure; it excites the nervous system and the vital activity of the individual more generally. In contact with the serum, phagocytosis is given a new force, whatever the illness concerned.[31]

The message that emerges from these overviews of contemporary knowledge concerning the action of the serum is that no one knew exactly how the serum worked, irrespective of their humoral or cellular inclinations. But what is significant is the widespread interest in having a convincing scientific explanation for the action of the serum. It was not sufficient, apparently, just to observe that serum worked; doctors—or more particularly the emerging groups of medical researchers—wanted to know why and how it worked. Of course, this is not an entirely new development; theories of drug action had already been elaborated in the seventeenth and eighteenth centuries bound into a range of experimental practices.[32] The older ones were, however, general theories and were not tied to specific drugs, nor did they mobilize microscopic observations let alone germ theories of disease.

While the debate around the mechanism of the serum's action was inconclusive, I think there are good reasons to think that this interest in serum's mode of action represents a significant innovation in pharmaceutical history. Indeed, I find the argument that this anticipates future developments in twentieth-century medicine more compelling than the claim that the statistical study of diphtheria's efficacy was a precursor to modern controlled clinical trials. The intense speculation and experimental research concerning how the serum functioned in the body represents something new particularly as applied to a specific medicine that targeted a single disease. This being said, I do not want to give the impression either that the laboratory research around serotherapy was completely new or that it was itself comparable to twentieth-century research on a number of grounds. Furthermore, reading the specialized press of the time, one does not get the impression that this fundamental scientific research interested the clinicians who were handling diphtheria and so it is hard to imagine that it ever exercised a direct influence on their choice of treatment.

The majority of the publications on the use of serum to treat diphtheria published in journals (both local and national, specialist and generalist) were given over to reports about doctors' personal clinical experience with the serum, without any reference to statistical arguments or more fundamental scientific research. The most common type of publication, particularly in local journals like the *Lyon médical* were quite detailed descriptions of the use of the serum on a few patients without any formal claim concerning their representativity. These articles translated into print an enthusiasm around the serum. But this enthusiasm was based on personal clinical experience rather than statistics or laboratory investigations. Indeed, this observation takes us back to a fundamental lesson in the history of science; we should not read past events in the light of the subsequent development of the science but make every effort to understand the position of the actors in terms of their own values and conceptions. Thus, we need to consider the culture of medical drugs at the time that serotherapy was introduced—the end of the nineteenth century. Browsing through any daily or weekly newspaper of the period, one is struck by the quantity of advertising for pharmaceutical products despite the fact that it was technically illegal to advertise medical drugs. Furthermore, these advertisements presented very general claims for the health benefits of the products without any apparent support for these claims. Let us take as an example an advertisement for Doctor Franck's 'health granules' (*Grains de santé*) that appeared in the *Revue Illustrée* of October 10, 1895. This advertisement is typical of those to be found in the generalist press selling a secret remedy to a very wide public.[33] The headline, Doctor Franck's Genuine Health Granules (*Véritables grains de santé de Docteur Franck*), sits above a drawing of two gentlemen talking; one is seated at a desk and wears glasses (presumable the eponymous Doctor Franck) and the other is wearing top hat and tails and carrying a cane. Under the picture we find the following copy.

> My dear client, take my *Grains de santé* they will cure your constipation, they will give you an appetite, they will bring you back sleep and gaity. You can hope to live to be a hundred years old like my old friend the wise man, who owes his longevity to these granules.

The basis of this promotional material was the implicit suggestion that other members of the public would benefit in the same way as Dr. Franck's 'old friend.' Such bold claims as curing constipation and prolonging the patient's life were backed up by the testimonials of satisfied customers almost always identified as men of standing: lawyers who had seen their pustules melt away or doctors describing the positive effects they had witnessed in their medical practice. Serotherapy was introduced into this world of Dr. Franck's Health Granules not into the modern world of drugs we are familiar with today where 'serious' products are tucked safely away behind the counter in sober bar-coded packages and are paid for through complex public or private health-insurance schemes. Today, the eye-catching dietary supplements or energy drinks are placed in a quite distinct marketing space from prescription drugs. In the nineteenth century there was, at the risk of understating the situation, considerable overlap. Furthermore, health products all depended on testimonials for establishing their reputation and for the confidence that patients placed in them. The corollary for doctors was the endorsement of a treatment as safe and effective by trustworthy colleagues. In the end, as I have suggested but cannot prove, the reason that serotherapy was adopted so widely in such a short period of time was largely thanks to old-fashioned mechanisms of word-of-mouth endorsement backed up by the national image of Emile Roux and the Pasteur Institute as serious and reliable purveyors of medical drugs. Serotherapy was also successful because it bound together a number of long-awaited elements into one product. It was a revolutionary treatment for a major disease, and was seen as being an effective cure emanating from a modern and successful science. Pasteur had on many occasions promised a therapeutic revolution based on the knowledge of microbes, and Roux, it seems, had delivered on this promise.[34]

In conclusion then, I want to underline the interpretation of efficacy in terms of the three elements that we have been exploring in this chapter; the statistical arguments, the mechanism of action and the testimonials based on clinical experience. It is common in medicine to consider the efficacy of a drug in precisely the opposite way. To imagine that there is some pre-determined efficacy (or lack of it) against a disease in an abstract, ideal organism and then to consider the different ways of determining the value of this property, preferably measuring it in precise figures. In this way, modern medicine has come to regard the clinical trial and its statistical analysis as the best measure of efficacy, with the elucidation of the mechanism as the explanation for this effect. The testimonial is seen to be a very unreliable indicator of any efficacy, but given the prominent role of opinion leaders in determining best clinical practices, it is difficult to dismiss it entirely. I believe that it is a historical error to place too much weight on the statistical arguments concerning the value of serotherapy, as it appears to me that personal clinical experience was still predominant in making up the minds of physicians at the end of the nineteenth century. But for the wider reflection about medical drugs as technological objects, we need to be aware of the shifting weights of these different elements, and it is clear that statistical arguments have become dominant over the second half of the twentieth century, at least in the official discourse.

NOTES

1. It is unsurprising that in the last 50 years the focus of technology studies has shifted from 'classical' machines to computers and communication devices. In light of the prominent place they occupy in modern life (at least for those with access to them) and the profound transformations they have wrought at home and in the workplace, we can well understand why they have attracted so much attention. See, for example, Sherry Turkle, *Alone Together: Why We Expect More from Technology and Less from Each Other* (New York: Basic Books, 2011).
2. Latour, Bruno 'Give me a laboratory and I will move the world' in Karin Knorr and Michael Mulkay (eds) *Science Observed*, (London: Sage, 1983), 141–70.
3. It is tempting to think of doping in these terms, but taking testosterone to improve one's performance in a cycling race is, to my mind, far from being the same thing as using a motorcycle to win. However 'augmented' they may be by the use of drugs, one's physical capacities remain one's physical capacities. I would argue that the addition of a mechanical prosthesis represents a more convincing frontier.

4. The idea of a deadly disease and its 'antidote' has traditionally been associated with thinking in terms of sympathy and harmony rather than machines or mechanics. Nevertheless, the idea that there might be a 'magic bullet' for each infectious disease orients us toward a more mechanistic vision of disease and pharmaceutical treatment. The term 'magic bullet' is associated with the name of Paul Ehrlich and his thinking of the action of medicines in terms of a 'lock and key' mechanism, another metaphor that lends support to a mechanical view of drug action.

5. Here I am referring to the mortality rate among people affected with the disease, not to be confused with the global mortality rate for the French population, for example, or the prevalence (or morbidity) which quantifies the proportion of a specified population that is affected by the disease in the first place.

6. It is tempting to suggest that the benefit/risk ratio is the pharmaceutical equivalent of mechanical advantage in classical physics while efficacy is closer to efficiency.

7. Today, the problem that is most often raised is the potential mismatch between a narrowly defined test population (determined by the inclusion and exclusion criteria for a clinical trial) versus the general population that an approved medication is used to treat. Thus, the absence of children and under-representation of women in clinical trials has been one of the points of attack in recent decades. This criticism does not even touch the thorny problem of off-label use, where a medical drug is prescribed for a clinical condition that has not even been the subject of clinical trials and so for which its efficacy remains undetermined. I will not even enter into the complex question of the placebo effect.

8. For more on standards in medicine and the foundations of evidence-based medicine, see Stefan Timmermans and Marc Berg, *The Gold Standard: The Challenge of Evidence-Based Medicine and Standardization in Health Care* (Philadelphia: Temple University Press, 2003).

9. This belief is translated into a demand for research on such biochemical mechanisms as part of the dossier that has to be completed in order to obtain an AMM (*Autorisation de mise sur le marché* – the official permit needed to sell a medical drug in France).

10. The FDA (the Food and Drug Administration) is the agency responsible for approving drugs in the US, and the EMA (European Medicines Agency, based, for the moment at least, in London) is the European equivalent, providing Europe-wide approval for drugs. Nevertheless, drugs are still approved in each member state of the European Union by its own national agency.

11. Gabriel Gachelin, 'The building up of a culture of standardization at the Institut Pasteur, 1885–1900.' *HAL*, web open archives, 2008, halshs-00335350.

12. These figures were widely circulated and often quoted. This report of Roux's intervention is from *La Semaine médicale*, vol. 14 no. 51, September 8, 1894, p. 407.

13. Louis Landouzy, *Les sérothérapies: leçons de thérapeutique et matière médicale, professées à la Faculté de Médecine de l'Université de Paris* (Paris: G. Carré et C. Naud, 1898), pp. 205–6.

14. Ibid, p. 208

15. Victor Chary, 'La mortalité par diphtérie en Europe avant et après l'application de la sérothérapie (étude statistique).' 1900. Thèse de médecine, Faculté de Médecine

de Paris. Jacques Bertillon was the brother of Alphonse Bertillon who introduced the use of anthropometry to the Paris police force. Jacques reformed the classification of causes of death in France.

16. This seems a particularly good year to choose, as there was a nationwide census in Britain in 1881, providing relatively reliable figures, at least in terms of the population of the country.

17. Louis Cobbett, 'Has antitoxine reduced the death rate from diphtheria in our large towns?' *Edinburgh Medical Journal*, 1900, pp. 521–47. The information concerning Liverpool, p. 531. While Cobbett himself was convinced of the utility of serotherapy in treating diphtheria, he nevertheless concluded by insisting on prophylactic hygiene measures as the best weapon available against the disease.

18. Anne Hardy, *The Epidemic Streets: Infectious Diseases and the Rise of Preventive Medicine 1856–1900*, (Oxford: Clarendon Press, 1993), p. 109.

19. Ibid, p. 82 ff.

20. While not markedly anti modern medicine, McKeown's argument was aimed at re-orienting the priorities of public health investment both in terms of research and applied public health measures. He argued that specific treatments and even vaccination (against smallpox, in particular) had only a very small influence on demographic shifts in the nineteenth century, and the real explanation for these changes was to be found in the rising standards of living in the wake of the industrial revolution. See Thomas McKeown, *Medicine in Modern Society* (London: George Allen and Unwin, 1965). The responses to his overall arguments have tended to focus on the specific question of the contribution of progress in medical science to life expectancy and mortality. See, for example, James Colgrove, 'The McKeown Thesis: A Historical Controversy and Its Enduring Influence' *American Journal of Public Health* 92, n° 5 (May 2002): 725–9.

21. The report of the use of serum in the diphtheria ward of the *Charité* hospital in Lyon suggests that patients were brought to the hospital for treatment and rarely received the serum prior to their arrival at the specialized ward. See Pierre Patet, 'La Sérothérapie à Lyon' (Lyon: Thesis for the Faculté de Médecine, 1895).

22. For more on the context in which Behring first proposed serotherapy, see Jonathan Simon, 'Emil Behring's Medical Culture: From Disinfection to Serotherapy,' *Medical History*, 51 (2007), 201–18.

23. See chapter 3 of the comprehensive history of immunology: Arthur Silverstein, *A History of Immunology* (San Diego: Academic Press, 1989).

24. Raymond Lemieux and Ulrike Spohr, 'How Emil Fischer Was Led to the Lock and Key Concept for Enzyme Specificity,' in *Advances in Carbohydrate Chemistry and Biochemistry* (San Diego: Academic Press, 1994), 1–19.

25. F. Himmelweit et al. (eds) *The collected papers of Paul Ehrlich*, (London: Pergamon, 1957), Vol. 3, p. 134.

26. Ibid, p. 135.

27. The most complete exploration of the differences between the research school around Louis Pasteur in Paris and that around Robert Koch in Berlin is to be found in Andrew Mendelsohn's Ph.D. thesis: John Andrew Mendelsohn, 'Cultures of

Bacteriology: Formation and Transformation of a Science in France and Germany, 1870–1914.' Ph.D. thesis, Princeton University, 1996.

28. Alfred I. Tauber and Leon Chernyak, *Metchnikoff and the Origins of Immunology: From Metaphor to Theory*, (Oxford: Oxford University Press, 1991).

29. Émile Roux and Louis Martin, 'Contribution à l'étude de la diphtérie (sérumthérapie)', *Annales de l'Institut Pasteur*, 8.9 (1894), 609–39. 'Sans vouloir traiter ici cette importante question doctrinale, nous dirons que le sérum antidiphtérique n'est pas antitoxique dans le sens propre du mot ; ajouté à la toxine il la laisse intacte ; injecté aux animaux il agit sur leurs cellules en les rendant, pour un temps comme insensibles au poison. . . .

'L'explication naturelle de ces faits n'est-elle pas dans l'action du sérum sur les cellules ? Les cellules bien vivaces des cobayes neufs répondent à la stimulation du sérum; chez les cobayes, aussi vigoureux en apparence, mais qui ont déjà été impressionnées par des produits microbiens, elles restent sans défense devant la toxine. L'étude de la réaction phagocytaire dans la diphtérie a été entreprise, à l'Institut Pasteur, par M. Gabritchevski; les constatations auxquelles il est arrivé s'accordent avec l'idée que les sérums préventifs sont stimulants et non antitoxiques.'

30. M. Funck, *Manuel de sérothérapie antidiphtérique* (Paris: Carré, 1895), p. 72.

31. Louis Landouzy, *Les sérothérapies: leçons de thérapeutique et matière médicale, professées à la Faculté de Médecine de l'Université de Paris* (Paris: G. Carré et C. Naud, 1898), p.188.

32. See Andreas-Holger Maehle, *Drugs on Trial: Experimental Pharmacology and Therapeutic Innovation in the Eighteenth Century* (Amsterdam: Rodopi, 1999) and for an earlier view on the same period, Melvin Earles, 'Early Theories of the Mode of Action of Drugs and Poisons,' *Annals of Science*, 17.2 (1961), 97–110.

33. Secret remedy was a legal category in France denoting a drug that did not figure in the official Pharmacopoeia and whose ingredients were not specified on the packaging. The sale of such drugs was illegal according to the 1803 pharmacy legislation, but was increasingly tolerated by the authorities.

34. For an analysis of Pasteur's success in terms of aligning his germ theory with traditional concerns in hygiene, see Bruno Latour's classic text; Bruno Latour, *The Pasteurization of France*. (Cambridge: Harvard University Press, 1993).

Chapter 5

Fitting Serum In

The Environment Shaping and Shaped by Serotherapy in France

In the previous chapter we explored the issue of how the serum was made to work. While the question of efficacy was at the center of our reflection, we were not looking retrospectively to determine the true efficacy of serotherapy as a treatment for diphtheria. This being said, it is not uncommon to hear the claim that the serum was the first such treatment to be truly effective. This position finds its corollary in the idea that before the introduction of the serum there was nothing that anyone could do for a patient suffering from diphtheria, an image of therapeutic impotence usually coupled with an attitude that any treatment before the serum must have been simple quackery. This belief in the effect of the serum and the dismissal of all its predecessors are part of the story that has coalesced around this particularly innovative product. We need to be careful when considering this kind of idealized history of the anti-diphtheria serum which places its discovery, development and use in a narrative of the progress of medical science that has become characteristic of the tales told about twentieth-century medicine. I hope that in the previous chapter we succeeded in showing how complex and unclear the issue of the efficacy of the serum turns out to be when examined closely. In this chapter we will be considering how serum shaped and was shaped by a number of factors in its environment, in particular the complementary technologies that developed around it, but also those that were displaced from the therapeutic space it came to occupy. This approach has the virtue of reminding us that the serum was not introduced into a therapeutic vacuum around diphtheria and that the new treatment had to establish a place on the hospital wards as well as in general practice.

EMBEDDING THE TECHNOLOGY

Inserted into multiple networks of distribution and consumption, the anti-diphtheria serum should not be considered as an independent stand-alone product ready for use. Instead it should be bound into a whole range of complementary objects and dispositions. Here we move beyond the classic image of a technological object as simply responding to a practical need and consider the context into which it is introduced. Again the aim is not just to see how the object adjusted to conform to a pre-existing situation but to examine how the object shapes its environment, and, at the same time, how this evolving environment is in return constitutive of the object. It is this extra step that aligns modern philosophers of technology, like Langdon Winner, Wiebe Bijker or Andrew Feenberg, all of whom have sought to bring the cultural and political implications of technology to the fore. [1] The political lesson is that technologies are not simply conceived to fit into a society, they are also active forces in shaping the society in which we live. This theme, very present in recent work on computing, video games and communication, will constitute a background element if not a leitmotif for the rest of this book. [2]

In this chapter our analysis of the serum moves beyond the production and distribution of the phials containing the product, but in a different direction from the last, showing how a space (both physical and conceptual) was fashioned for this new medical drug. This takes us closer to the rich, although incompletely documented life of the serum in French society. Nevertheless this is only a start, as this examination of the immediate context of serotherapy fails to take into account a number of key considerations necessary for understanding the form and functioning of the serum in a specific historical, political, and national context. In the chapters that follow we will address the cultural and political features of the serum and its manufacture in their own right, considering in particular the political and juridical aspects of the serum and serotherapy as it was introduced in France's Third Republic. In the present chapter, we will look at the lower-level practical considerations that concerned the diagnosis and care of diphtheria on hospital wards and in doctors' offices around France. We will do this in three sections, a first one dealing with the modes of administration of the drug, a second one treating the rise of the bacteriological diagnosis of the disease and its links to serotherapy, and a third section on the alternative treatments for diphtheria available at the time the serum was introduced in France.

ASSOCIATED TECHNOLOGIES

How then did the modes of diagnosis and care of diphtheria change following the introduction of the serum? We have already seen in some detail how serum was extracted from a horse and placed in a glass phial with its immunization

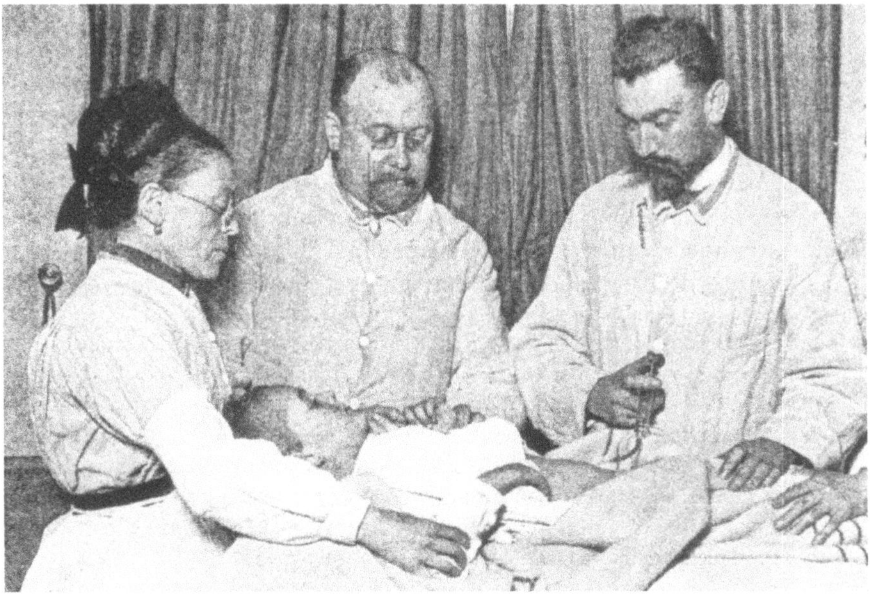

Figure 5.1 Detail from a photograph illustrating the use of the serum (Figure 7.2). *Figaro Illustré*, vol 12, no. 56, November 1894. Private collection, photograph by the author.

power marked on a label, the figure being based on the all-important evaluation procedure employing toxin (produced by the cultivation of diphtheria bacteria) and guinea pigs. Although there is little surviving information beyond the bare production figures, we know that these phials of serum were sent out all over France from the Pasteur Institute.[3] The packages were shipped to doctors, to pharmacies (relatively few, it appears), but mostly to the Prefectures, the administrative centers located in every department, and then redistributed to hospitals and the *bureaux de bienfaisance*[4] (see Figure 3.2).

Let us start, then with a very obvious technology closely bound to the clinical use of the serum—the syringe. The intraperitoneal injection of 10 or 20 cubic centimeters of the serum required an unusually large syringe, and an extended delivery tube.

In the feature story for *Le Figaro*'s illustrated supplement on the diphtheria serum that appeared in November 1894, the injection of serum using a large syringe figured prominently in one of the photographs (Figure 5.1). While syringes had been in use in medicine in France at least since the 1850s, it was rare to have to inject such large quantities of a liquid into any patient. Indeed, syringe manufacturers seized the opportunity to launch a new range of products designed specifically for this use.

Emile Roux found himself directly involved in the marketing of these syringes, as manufacturers played on the close association between the Pasteur Institute (and Roux's name in particular) and the anti-diphtheria serum. The following example of an advertisement by a certain Brenot, manufacturer of surgical instruments, comes from Roux's own papers, and is very likely drawn from a larger dossier containing Roux's complaints against such manufacturers. Indeed, Roux resisted what he saw as the commercial exploitation of the Pasteur Institute's achievements, asking Marcel Mérieux, for example, not to cite the name of the Institute in his advertisements for the private microbiological diagnosis service he launched in Lyon. Returning to Brenot's advertisement, under the headline 'Sterilisable syringe for the injection of Dr. Roux's antidiphteric serum' we can read the following copy:

> The marvellous discovery of the antidiphtheria serum by Dr. ROUX requires a perfect syringe whose parts are easy to sterilise. I was in a better position than anyone else to construct a special model answering to the needs of this new and admirable application of sub-cutaneous injection.
>
> I also have the advantage of being able to inform you by means of this note that my model was chosen over all the others for the injections of Dr. Roux's serum, and it is now used at the Pasteur Institute and in diverse diphtheria services in the Paris hospitals.[5]

Despite Roux's objections, the temptation for businessmen to use his name was just too great, and there was not a great deal that he could do about it, particularly in the case of syringe manufacturers outside France.

But syringes were not the only technologies mobilized in the integration of serum into contemporary medical practices. Another central technology that has been mentioned but not yet examined in any detail is that of microbiological diagnosis, which was intimately linked to both the deployment and the acceptance of serotherapy, although not in the most direct or obvious manner. Looking at the place of the microscope in the clinical handling of diphtheria helps us to contextualize serotherapy in terms of the much wider movement around the establishment of pathological microbiology in Europe at the end of the nineteenth century.

Diphtheria was one of a number of infectious diseases for which microbiologists succeeded in identifying a bacterium thought to be responsible for the disease. This was one of the characteristic achievements of the movement dominated by the schools of Louis Pasteur in France and Robert Koch in Germany, with the discovery of the eponymous Koch bacillus responsible for tuberculosis marking the highpoint in this pioneering period of medical microbiology. Thus, the reader needs to bear this context in mind, as the much wider impact of this movement had a bearing on the significance of its application to diphtheria. This point should become clearer when we discuss the more general questions arising from the microbiological transformation of the diagnosis of diphtheria. Nevertheless, before examining this issue we need first to understand the history of the diagnosis of the disease, both bacteriological and clinical.

CULTURES FOR CLASSIFICATION

In the race to identify the microbial causal agents of infectious diseases at the end of the nineteenth century, the credit for identifying the bacterium responsible for diphtheria is generally shared between Edwin Klebs and Friedrich Löffler. Klebs observed the bacterium in 1883, but it was Löffler who cultivated and characterized it, suggesting in his publication on the *Corynebacterium diphtheriae* that the lethal nature of the disease was due to a toxin produced by the bacillus.[6] In 1888, Alexandre Yersin and Emile Roux succeeded in separating the toxin from the bacteria by using a ceramic filter designed by Charles Chamberland. While the isolation of the toxin would become important in the production of the serum, as we have already seen, it was the identification of the characteristic bacteria that would have the greatest impact on the destiny of diphtheria as a disease. The technique of culturing throat samples (the samples were normally taken directly from the false membrane that formed in the throat of a victim of the disease) and then observing the characteristic corynebacterium (this name was chosen because of the bacterium's knotted rod shape) brought about a number of significant changes. First, this microbiological diagnosis redefined the disease, opening up the possibility of its bacteriological identification rather than relying on the characteristic clinical symptoms of the disease. This, as we shall see in more detail below, was a double transformation of the disease; first, the microbiological technique offered a new means for identifying diphtheria, and second, and more importantly in the long term, the isolation of the bacteria responsible for the disease opened the way for a reconceptualization of the nature of the disease itself. For converts to the new bacteriology, diphtheria was no longer to be considered a collection of symptoms explained in principle by some underlying pathological lesion but the result of the action of an invading microorganism. What's more, this particular bacillus produced a lethal toxin, adding another layer to the image of the pathogenic invader profiting from the victim's inattention in order to penetrate into the body and lay it low. The multiplication of the bacillus in the body not only threatened to disrupt vital functions on the model of other bacilli, but the Corynebacterium went further, producing a toxin powerful enough to kill its host.

As a corollary to the profound transformations ushered in by Löffler's work, this new technique of microbiological diagnosis also contributed to the statistical success of serotherapy, as we discussed in detail in the preceding chapter. But perhaps most significantly of all, this technique applied to diphtheria as well as tuberculosis and other infectious diseases, would radically change the perception of the medical doctor at the turn of the century. I will return to this wider influence of microbiology on the medical profession at the end of this section, but first I want to consider how this technology transformed the nature of diphtheria itself, and the effect this in turn had on the statistics concerning the disease.

One way of engaging this issue is by way of the mortality figures we were considering in the previous chapter. Indeed, those who sought to compile these figures, often with the goal of assessing the value of serotherapy in the treatment of diphtheria, were confronted with particularly thorny problems concerning the classification of the disease and those considered close to it. When presenting the figures in the previous chapter I simply passed over this very real problem in silence. Put succinctly, the question is: when different people counted cases of diphtheria, were they really counting the same things? The differences of opinion are particularly clear if we try to compare the statistics concerning the disease produced in different national contexts governed by different diagnostic traditions. These differences in opinion make it difficult to answer an important and apparently straightforward question—how many people died from diphtheria in the second half of the nineteenth century? Trying to respond to this question leads us into a lengthy digression, but one that will in turn raise a number of important issues related to the analysis of the disease.

Returning to Chary's medical thesis, we can now go a little further into the details of the comparative diphtheria mortality rates in Paris (9.9 per 10,000) and London (1.7 per 10,000) for 1881. In making these calculations, Chary was confronted with the difficult problem of nomenclature. When considering the different causes of death proposed in the nineteenth century, what was he to include as diphtheria? The problem was particularly acute for the cases classified as 'croup' either side of the channel. The British had tended to count croup apart from diphtheria while the French had, since the eighteenth century, increasingly placed croup in the same category as diphtheria. But it is not at all clear that the French and British doctors had exactly the same conception of what croup was, and this national difference of opinion was just one factor in divergent diagnostic criteria often attributable to personal sensibilities as much as to medical preconceptions. While Chary did have clear views on the question, and an idea of the appropriate statistical strategy to adopt, this did not render the comparison between the two countries any more reliable.

> The question remains of knowing what has been designated by the terms 'croup' and 'diphtheria.' As for the latter, there is, in the context of the time-period that we have chosen [1880–1900], almost no doubt, as diphtheria was already a clinically defined disease. Things were different for croup. Diphtheritic croup along with other types of croup and laryngitis were gathered together under the same rubric for a long time in England. Here [in France] the dominant tendency was to reserve the name 'croup' for diphtheritic laryngitis, and, in the statistics, croup progressively changed place.[7]

Thus, the British tended to count all forms of croup apart from diphtheria, and lump the condition in with other, generally benign, throat diseases. In France, while certain forms of croup were not considered 'diphtheritic,' those that were became increasingly frequently included in the statistics as cases of diphtheria. This meant that the same case of 'diphtheritic croup,' a disease clinically much closer to diphtheria than common laryngitis, could well be counted in with benign throat infections in Britain and be assimilated to diphtheria in France. This difference in classification evidently had an impact on the statistics in the two countries, as equivalent epidemiological situations would automatically result in a higher absolute mortality rate in France (because more deaths would be attributed to diphtheria) but a lower relative mortality rate with respect to the number of cases of diphtheria (because many more cases would be considered to be diphtheria in France than in Britain).

Nevertheless, the problem of classification was not limited to the differential distribution of sets of symptoms between croup and diphtheria in different national traditions. To enter a little deeper into the complexity of the debates over the identification of diphtheria, I want to consider four different names that were in use in the eighteenth and nineteenth centuries in France. These names are *angine couenneuse*, *angine gangréneuse*, *croup* and *diphtérie*, which can be literally translated into English as leathery angina, gangrenous angina, croup and diphtheria. In order to make sense of these multiple denominations in the national clinical context, however, I will use the French names. While initially directing our attention to the principal symptoms of the disease, an examination of these different names allows us to chart the uncertain boundaries of the disease. This multiplication of names reinforces the argument that diphtheria was not a well-defined condition with a general consensus among practicing doctors as to which of their patients suffered from the disease. Furthermore, while some doctors used the terms indifferently, for many doctors each term designated a specific disease, albeit one they might disagree over.

ANGINE COUENNEUSE VERSUS *GANGRÉNEUSE*

In French, *angine* is a general term for an inflamed, painful sore throat usually accompanied by difficulty in swallowing and sometimes even difficulty breathing, a common (and often benign) complaint that was not to be confused with diphtheria. Nevertheless, diphtheria was to be suspected when the sore throat was accompanied by discoloration around the tonsils (and, in particular, the presence of distinctive white patches in this area) or, more characteristically, when a membrane started to form in the larynx. This 'false membrane,' skin or rind, as it is expressed in the adjective *couenneuse*, could be fatal, causing suffocation by obstructing the patient's trachea or windpipe. Once the trachea was completely closed by the membrane, air could no longer reach the patient's lungs and he or she would suffocate. Thus, *angine couenneuse* points to the false membrane as the characteristic symptom, and many believed that the absence of such a membrane was sufficient to disqualify a case as being diphtheria. The adjective *gangréneuse*, however, turns our attention away from the 'false membrane' and toward the necrosis of the affected region; the medical definition of gangrene being the 'complete destruction of life in one part of the body, with vital reactions conserved in the adjoining parts.'[8] That the characteristic symptom might be the appearance of a membrane or a localized necrosis opens the way for disagreement between specialists, in particular concerning the necessity of a false membrane for the diagnosis of diphtheria.

Suffocation due to the spreading of the false membrane to block the windpipe was heralded by the victim's increasing difficulty in breathing, and the word 'croup,' which exists in both English and French, is thought to derive from the gasping noise that children made as a membrane progressively restricted the passage of air toward the lungs. Thus, the term croup takes us back to the false membrane, evoking the suffocation that could kill the patient. This kind of death was particularly dramatic, although the powerful toxic effect of diphtheria was even more redoubtable, with victims often dying suddenly of a heart attack when they appeared to be well on the road to recovery. Nevertheless, as we have already seen, the British considered croup to be a different disease from diphtheria, in particular following the contributions of the Scottish doctor Francis Home. Indeed, the word croup had its origins as a local Scottish term, probably onomatopoeic as I suggested above. Ironically, Home himself does not propose this vernacular term for a disease that he believed he was the first to identify.

> As this disease has different vulgar names, for I am told, that on the west coast, they call it the *Chock*, or *Stuffing*, a technical one becomes absolutely necessary. A name is best given from the apparent symptoms, which are always conspicuous, while the cause is generally hidden, and often doubtful. The leading symptoms here, are, the shrill voice, and difficult breathing. It, therefore, may properly be called *Suffocatio stridula*.[9]

For Home, then, the difficulty in breathing is presented as the characteristic symptom of croup as distinct from diphtheria. Diphtheria, he believed, was a much more general systemic disease in which suffocation was incidental, while croup was signified by a particular form of suffocation. It is, of course, paradoxical that Home should leave a lasting trace on the reporting of this disease in Britain by differentiating the disease known by the common name for croup, while the descriptive Latin binomial term (reflecting botanical nomenclature) he found more suitable, *Suffocatio stridula*, was never adopted.

We turn now to the last of the four terms, *diphtérie*, which was—under this particular denomination—a peculiarly nineteenth-century malady. The disease found its classic clinical definition in the work of a French doctor, Pierre Bretonneau early in the century. In a memoir presented in 1821 before the Royal Academy of Medicine in Paris, he outlined the characteristics of *la phlegmasie dipthéritique* or diphtheria. Indeed, Bretonneau is generally credited with having introduced the term 'diphtheria,' derived from a Greek word for leather (*diphthera*), although he used it mostly as an adjective, *diphtérique* or *diphtéritique*. The 1821 memoir was published along with others in 1826 under the title *Traité de la diphthérite*, which would serve as a reference for the clinical definition of the disease throughout the century. Bretonneau's work consisted in a detailed study of angina in adults and children, followed by generalizations from these observations aimed at characterizing a number of diseases. Indeed, he saw himself as confronting a double problem: first, the confusion of a number of distinct diseases under the same name and, second, the identification of a number of different diseases where there was really only one.

Bretonneau's choice of the term diphtheria once again draws our attention to the leathery false membrane, and he did pay particular attention to the membrane and the discoloration of the tonsils. Nevertheless, Bretonneau did not consider the false membrane an indispensable feature of the disease.

This preliminary detour around the various terms in use in the nineteenth century gives us an idea of the confused and confusing diagnostic territory into which the microbiological test was introduced.

The 1880s saw the publication of a major medical reference work in France, the multivolume *Dictionnaire Encyclopédique des sciences médicales*. This extensive work provided the space for specialists to go into detail concerning their field of medicine. In the entry on *diphthérie* (the spelling of *diphtérie* in French was variable as well) dating from 1884, Albert Sanné summarized the state of the art in the following terms.[10]

> Disease—general, specific, infectious, contagious—having as its principal objective characteristic the production of fibrous exsudations on the mucous membranes or on the profound layer of the epidermis. These are customarily designated by the term false membranes.[11]

Thus, while he mentioned the various approaches to the disease, and in particular the path followed by the British under the influence of Home, Sanné stuck to the false membrane as characteristic of the disease, although admitting it was not essential for making a positive diagnosis. Just a few years later, in 1889, Jules Simon would offer quite a different definition of diphtheria. We have already encountered the head of the diphtheria ward at the hospital for sick children in Paris who allowed Roux to test his new serum. In a series of lectures on the disease, Dr. Simon leaves no room for doubt; for him, diphtheria is now a disease identified with the presence of a characteristic microbe.

> Diphtheria has its specific baccilus; any false membrane that contains this microorganism is diphtheritic, any false membrane that does not contain it is not due to diphtheria.[12]

Simon was expressing an increasingly widespread view. For the generation of Pastorian doctors who believed in the specific pathogen as the explanation for infectious disease (and possibly for non-infectious diseases as well), the only real diagnostic question was the identity of the pathogen. Thus, the isolation of a bacterium considered responsible for the disease changed the terms of diagnostic debate, although it did not put an end to all discussion.

DIPHTHERIA UNDER THE MICROSCOPE

In their handbook on microbiology, the *Précis de microbie*, first published in the same year as Jules Simon's definition cited above, Léon-Henri Thoinot and E.-Jules Masselin do not adopt quite such a categorical position. They present the clinical symptoms and characteristics of diphtheria as the means for diagnosing the disease. Although the book is about microbiology, it is only in certain circumstances that doctors should engage with the task of culturing the bacillus. Thus, while the title of the book clearly places them in the Pastorian school of Emile Roux, when it comes to defining the disease the authors present an inventory of its clinical manifestations.

> Human diphtheria is characterized anatomically and clinically by a false membrane that is most often found on the tonsils and the uvula (*diphthérie pharyngée*, *angine diphthéritique*). The false membrane can also occupy diverse sections of the respiratory passages: larynx (*croup* or *diphthérie layngée*); nasal sinuses (*coryza diphthéritique*); trachea, bronchial tubes (*trachéite*, *bronchite* and *broncho-pneumonie diphthéritiques*); it can also occur on the mucous membranes of the mouth, of the vagina or on the conjunctiva, as well as any uncovered surface of the skin (*diphthérie cutanée*). A most serious condition, diphtheria can kill mechanically (for example, *diphthérie laryngée* or *croup*), but it kills most often by intoxication: the patient is poisoned by the condition.[13]

Before any discussion of the microbe that they considered to be the cause of the disease, Thoinot and Masselin limit themselves to the superficially observable symptoms of diphtheria. Nevertheless, as the title of the work already tells us, their goal is to communicate the new science of 'microbie' with all the relevant techniques for modern medicine. They recommend the cultivation of a throat swab on a solid medium of peptonized serum from cows, sheep or horses.[14] Four years later, they published a second edition of their book with a lot of additional information. For the best results, a medium of 'gelatinized serum' should be kept at 33–37°C; in these conditions the diphtheria bacillus would multiply rapidly giving colonies that would be clearly visible around the lines of 'seeding' within a day.

The second edition of the book, with its title changed to focus attention on the techniques involved in microbiological medical diagnosis, also contains specific advice concerning the best coloring techniques not featured earlier. Here, the authors recommend Emile Roux's technique for staining the sample, using methyl green and violet from the dahlia.

Thanks in large part to practical manuals like the one by Thoinot and Masselin, as well as the course in 'Microbie' taught by Emile Roux and Louis Martin at the Institut Pasteur in Paris, more and more doctors were becoming capable of performing bacteriological diagnostic tests. In Lyon, for example, Francois Rabot, who was in charge of the diphtheria ward at the *Charité* hospital—the *salle St Jeanne*—organized a team for culturing and identifying known pathogenic microbes. One of the sisters on the ward specialized in taking samples from the patients' false membranes, while 'Brother Seyve' headed up Rabot's artisanal on-site laboratory. Here he cultured and examined the specimens.[15] Thus, starting in the 1890s, the clinical diagnosis of diphtheria was being complemented by such tests in an increasing number of settings, giving the disease a new dimension. The disease confirmed by a positive microbiological test was increasingly referred to as 'true diphtheria.' Thus, this rise in microbiological diagnosis sidestepped the complexity of clinical diagnosis that I presented above. In celebratory readings of the rise of microbiology, the diagnosis by microscopic observation of bacteria provided the solution to the diagnostic problems not only for diphtheria but for other infectious diseases like tuberculosis as well. The disease became identified with its causal agent, and so the clinical symptoms became secondary. But this vision is premised on a rather superficial reading of the history of microbiological diagnosis. While it did add an important and potentially consensual element to the clinician's art, this technique also introduced its own problems and ambiguities.

In the case of diphtheria, there was a particular problem of which the researchers were only too aware, the presence of the bacillus responsible for diphtheria in healthy subjects. While some advanced the solution of the healthy carrier, the extent of the bacillus did not seem to support this idea.[16] Another confusing observation was that the bacillus did not always provoke 'experimental diphtheria' in animals either. Certain strains could be inoculated into sensitive animals like guinea pigs without provoking similar symptoms to human diphtheria.

Nevertheless, the issue of the nature of disease and diagnosis at the end of the nineteenth century goes much deeper than technical issues over the presence or absence of the bacillus in healthy or sick individuals. There is a more general observation to make that applies to other diseases besides diphtheria. Most doctors, even the most convinced believers in microbial pathogens, did not think of diseases in term of the presence of such pathogens. A disease, and consequently its diagnosis, was understood in terms of a group of characteristic symptoms. Even if an increasing number of doctors thought that the pathogen caused the disease, this did not mean that they equated the disease with the bacillus, far from it. This profound ontological shift would take at least another half a century. Nevertheless, since the 1940s this identification has become such a commonplace that it is hard for today's doctors to see how it could have been otherwise, particularly once the profession had admitted the role of microbes in causing certain diseases. Consequently, today it seems evident that the laboratory test should be regarded as *the* diagnostic tool, with clinical symptoms falling into the secondary role of orienting the doctor toward the most appropriate test. Diagnosis is bound to etiology, with clinical symptoms constituting secondary phenomena that help to reveal the true cause. In this configuration, however, it is only the confirmation of the presence of the cause that permits the definitive diagnosis.

This profound transformation in modern medicine—the heart of the Pastorian revolution—has not been without loss for the medical doctor. While the reliance on microscopes and laboratory technique has been an integral part of the promotion of scientific medicine after the Second World War, it has demanded a sacrifice on the part of the medical profession itself. The subtlety and complexity of clinical diagnosis has always served the interests of the medical profession, and at the end of the nineteenth century doctors already saw what they risked in placing too much emphasis on the bacteriological test. The development of the authority of laboratory tests would be at the expense of the authority and liberty of the physician. This new relationship negotiated between the clinician and the laboratory in its multiple aspects would of course constitute one of the greatest changes in the medical profession over the twentieth century. A detailed discussion of what was at stake, although interesting, takes us too far from the question at hand, which is the importance of microbiological technologies in integrating the serum. Before turning to a reflection on how the serum fitted in with these new techniques,

I would like to quote Michael Worboys's conclusion from his study of the bacteriological revolution in Britain at the turn of the century. Although specifically about the situation in Britain, it nevertheless gives a good overview of the central role of bacteriology in the transformation of medicine in this period.

> By 1900, bacteriology represented above all the conversion of medicine and surgery to specific aetiological and pathological understandings of disease. This change was not wholly the product of bacteriology; developments in physiology, therapeutics and other medical specialisms had also moved medicine in the same direction. The new models of disease were not constructed entirely in mechanistic, reductionist terms, nor were ontological conceptions of disease dominant. Doctors did think more in terms of causes, and tried to relate causes to effects, but there were differences by area of work, age, training, interests and, no doubt, personal inclination. In no case did doctors construct causes or effects as simple and direct. The most decisive change was not the establishment of specific aetiological and pathological models, though certain exemplars structured expectations; rather, it was the spread of the assumption that the mechanisms of disease ought to be knowable and demonstrable, and that such an understanding would open the path to more effective preventive and curative interventions. This was a vision that both followed and fed the changing identity of the medical profession as an increasingly competent and effective expert body whose science-based work served both individual patients and society as a whole.[17]

DIAGNOSIS AND SEROTHERAPY

We turn now to more specific questions related to the bacteriological diagnosis of diphtheria and the introduction of the serotherapy; the effects of this diagnosis on statistics and the integration of such tests into the treatment of patients. While it is impossible to say in detail how this new form of diagnosis affected the statistics on the lethality of diphtheria, we see its effects regularly in publications on the question. Thus for example, Emile Roux already re-worked his statistics on the diphtheria ward at the *Hôpital des Enfants-Malades* in Paris for his presentation in Budapest in terms of the microbial determination of the disease.

> These are the raw statistics [for these figures, see page 54], but to correctly evaluate the question we need to subtract from the 448 children admitted to the diphtheria ward the 128 who were not infected with diphtheria due to the Klebs-Löffler bacilli as was revealed by bacteriological examination. We should subtract a further 20 children who died before any treatment could be given. This leaves 300 cases of true diphtheria with 78 deaths or 26%, while the statistics from the prior period based on the same conditions give a mortality rate of 50%.[18]

Roux's revised calculations based on the results of microbiological diagnosis only changed the mortality rates by a couple of percentage points and in this case the proposed revision was not in favor of the serum. Be that as it may, we can already see from this example how the alignment of 'true diphtheria' with the identification of a specifc bacillus (in this case the *Corynebacterium diphtheriae* bacterium) under the microscope has the capacity to transform these statistics one way or the other. We can also observe an even more direct relationship between serotherapy and microbiological diagnostic techniques in the pages of the specialized press starting in 1894. Following Roux's announcement in Budapest, advertisements started to appear for microbiological diagnosis services. Thus, the December 1894 issue of *Le Bulletin médical* carried the following advertisement for a diagnostic kit.

> Kit from the *Presse médicale*, prepared by Adrian and co., Paris. Giving the right to a free diagnosis of diphtheria.
>
> This kit—for medical doctors only—contains two tubes of getalinised serum, a sterilised glass tube, a spatula for seeding [the bacteria], instructions on how to use the kit and a pre-printed return envelope to 'The Presse médicale Laboratory,' 3 Rue Racine, Paris, which will make the diagnosis for free within 24 hours and will then send out the results. The price of the kit is 3 francs and it can be found in any pharmacy.[19]

This advertisement was placed opposite an article where Dr. Moizard from the *Hôpital Trousseau* in Paris reported another set of positive results for the use of the serum.[20] While the diagnosis (delivered within 24 hours) is offered free of charge, the kit cost 3 francs, the same price as the anti-diphtheria serum itself. Although such diagnostic tests had been available for a number of years, the arrival of serotherapy opened up substantial new markets for these products.

As the Belgian specialist Dr. Funck pointed out in 1898 there were now four reasons to carry out this microbiological diagnosis. First, such tests would help to provide accurate statistics concerning the disease and its treatment, notably its treatment using serotherapy. Indeed, he estimated that a quarter of diagnoses based purely on clinical symptoms were incorrect. Second, to improve prophylaxis by knowing which patients to isolate, and third for prognosis; to determine the veritable danger posed by a particular case. Last, but not least, Funck claimed that the tests were necessary for treatment, precisely because of their specific nature. From the perspective of treatment, the generalization of these microbiological exams could permit the timely introduction of a specific treatment but only where one could reasonably expect its universally acknowledged curative effects; that is to say in the case where the Löffler bacillus played the principal role in the disease state.[21]

Thus, an increasing interest in combinations of pathogenic bacteria found by the systematic use of the microscope promised to turn serotherapy into a completely effective specific treatment for 'true' diphtheria, where the Löffler bacteria existed in isolation. The rise in demands for such tests, whether provided by the doctors or hospitals themselves like the one maintained by Rabot at the *Charité* in Lyon, or by external services, such as the one set up by Marcel Mérieux upon his return to Lyon from Paris, reflects a rise in this way of thinking about infectious diseases. This whole movement was important on a number of levels, and it would be an error to limit our vision of microbiological tests as simply a new diagnostic tool. The use of the microscope had a strong symbolic force, serving to divide the ancients from the moderns in turn-of-the-century medical practice.

Before serotherapy, which was a specific treatment meant to neutralize precisely the toxin-producing Klebs-Löffler bacteria, testing for the bacillus was justified in terms of hygienic intervention. The presence of the bacteria, it was argued, confirmed that there was the potential for a contagious epidemic, and the appropriate steps needed to be taken. Nevertheless, prior to serotherapy, a positive test would have little effect on the therapeutic approach when compared to a clinical identification of diphtheria based on the 'classic' symptoms. Following the introduction of the serum, however, many doctors considered that the treatment would only work against 'true' diphtheria, and so knowing that the bacillus was present could serve as an invaluable guide to the appropriate therapy. More importantly, in the absence of the bacillus, the serum was considered useless.

While in principle this analysis makes sense, in practice the decision to use the serum was usually taken before the results of the test could be known. It took at least 24 hours to cultivate a throat sample for inspection, and yet, as we can see in this manual by Georges Lemière from 1895, experts agreed that for the best prognosis, the serum had to be administered as soon as possible.

> As soon as a child is affected by a complaint that might be diphtheria, whether the diagnosis is certain or possible, inject him subcutaneously with 20 cc of antitoxic serum then immediately seek to establish a precise diagnosis. There is only one way to do so and that is to perform a bacteriological diagnosis which requires twenty-four hours and, except in urgent cases—asphyxiating children or those who appear intoxicated—one should await the result of this bacteriological exam before continuing or stopping the treatment. But, and we cannot insist too much on this point, the treatment needs to be started as soon as possible. This is understandable in a disease where death comes by intoxication, one needs to act while there is as little poison in the blood as possible.[22]

Thus, faced with the exigency of having to start the serotherapy as soon as possible the microbiological analysis could only play a role in the decision about whether or not to continue the treatment. The logic was that the serum, as a specific medicine, should only be used in cases of infection with the corynebacterium, and some doctors even went as far as recommending that the serum not be used when staphylococcus was found to be present along with the diphtheria bacillus. But if the serum had to be used before the physician could obtain the results of the test, then one can legitimately question the utility of these bacteriological tests. Rather than acting as a guide to prescriptive practice, they were part of the general integration of the serum into a larger bacteriological framework. While they could not be used to determine the treatment, they could be integrated into a subsequent statistical analysis, providing data for better understanding the disease as a bacteriological phenomenon.[23] But most important for the present analysis, inserting the serotherapy into the surrounding context of bacteriological tests gave a place and a sense to both the developing microbiological laboratory practices and to the serum itself. As we will be arguing in the following chapters, the perception of serum was to a large extent informed by precisely these associations.

THERAPIES BEFORE SEROTHERAPY

To conclude this chapter, we would like briefly to recall a fundamental point that is often overlooked in the history of medical innovation; serotherapy was far from being the only possible treatment for diphtheria when it was introduced across France in 1895. While many doctors simply refrained from any therapeutic intervention in face of a diagnosis of diphtheria, there was a range of different approaches available for handling the disease in the second half of the nineteenth century, particularly in the hospital setting. Tracheotomy, following its promotion by Bretonneau, had become widespread in this period, notably to prevent suffocation by the membrane that formed in the throat. In the 1880s, tracheotomy was increasingly replaced by 'intubation' using a whole range of specialized surgical equipment designed for this purpose. This technique involved inserting a metal tube through the membrane, allowing the patient to breathe through the tube. One of these systems for inserting tubes through the membrane, the O'Dwyer tube was particularly favored in France, and looking at the history of what happened in the hospitals in Lyon, we see that it was widely used in the 1880s. Nevertheless, it seems that by the 1890s, Rabot, in his diphtheria ward at the *Hospices Civils* was trying to limit the use of intubation as much as possible due to infections associated with the tube being left in the patient's throat for a relatively long time. Rabot recommended instead the use of opium and topical disinfection applied directly to the membrane in the hope that young patients would recover before any more radical (surgical) intervention was needed.

In a medical thesis defended in Paris in 1893 (again, just prior to the introduction of the serotherapy) Eugène Aschkinazi reviewed the different methods used for treating diphtheria. We can see from his presentation that there was a general feeling that specialists had more or less identified the appropriate response, with the different treatments all based on the same principle. The preferred method involved the topical disinfection of the membrane with adjuvant use of surgery (tracheotomy or intubation) when necessary, and so Aschkinazi's review comes down to an inventory of the different disinfectants used. While the author oriented his study toward the promotion of his preferred product, '*stérésol*,' [24] the review nevertheless serves as a reminder that serotherapy was not introduced into a therapeutic vacuum. Although we have no way of knowing which products were used where and in what quantities, we need to bear in mind the displacement of these established treatments that the success of serotherapy implied. In the next chapter we will put forward an argument as to how and why the serum managed to displace these alternatives in a relatively short space of time.

NOTES

1. See, for example, Wiebe E. Bijker, *Of Bicycles, Bakelites, and Bulbs: Toward a Theory of Sociotechnical Change*. (Cambridge MA: The MIT Press, 1997).

2. Sherry Turkle, *The Second Self: Computers and the Human Spirit*. (Cambridge MA: The MIT Press, 2005).

3. The distribution of the serum from the Pasteur Institute was initially limited to Paris, but starting in early 1895, production levels were sufficient to supply the needs across France. We will have more to say about this issue of national distribution of serum in subsequent chapters.

4. The prefecture is the administrative center of a French department. The prefect of a department was appointed by the government, rather than being an elected official and was responsible for enforcing centrally established law and order. Hence, they made a good relay for national projects like this as they did not 'suffer' from potentially disruptive local allegiances.

5. Advertisement by Brenot, a Paris instrument manufacturer. Archives of the Institut Pasteur.

6. Friedrich Loeffler, 'Untersuchung über die Bedeutung der Mikroorganismen für die Entstehung der Diphtherie' *Mitteilungen des kaiserlichen Gesundheitsamtes* 2 (1884) 421–499.

7. Victor Chary, 'La mortalité par diphtérie en Europe avant et après l'application de la sérothérapie (étude statistique).' 1900. Thèse de médecine, 'Faculté de Médecine' de Paris, p. 13 'Il s'agit encore de savoir ce qu'on a désigné sous les noms croup et diphtérie. Quant à la dernière, il n'y a presque pas de doute : dans les

limites du temps que nous avons pris, la diphtérie était déjà une maladie cliniquement définie. Il en était autrement avec le croup. Le croup diphtérique et les autres croups, autres laryngites, étaient longtemps réunis sous la même rubrique en Angleterre. La tendance à réserver le nom croup pour les laryngites diphtérique a prévalue ici, et dans la statistique, le croup changeait progressivement sa place.'

8. Émile Littré, *Dictionnaire de la langue française* (2nd edition, 1872–1877) Gangrène—Terme de médecine. Destruction complète de la vie dans une partie du corps, avec conservation de la réaction vitale dans les parties contiguës.

9. Francis Home, *An Inquiry into the Nature, Cause, and Cure of the Croup* (Edinburgh, 1765), p. 34.

10. The actual publication date is soon after Löffler's work which is not mentioned at all. It is probable that the article was prepared well beforehand, as the dictionary started to be published in 1879.

11. Albert Sanné, 'Diphthérie' in A. Dechambre (dir.) *Dictionnaire Encyclopédique des sciences médicales*, vol. 29 (DIA-DIU) (Paris: Asselin & Masson, 1884), p. 548. Maladie générale, spécifique, infectieuse, contagieuse, ayant pour caractère objectif principal la production, sur les muqueuses ou sur la couche profonde de l'épiderme, d'exsudations fibrineuses designees habituellement sous le nom de fausses membranes. Ignorée pendant des siècles, en tant que maladie générale, la diphthérie n'était connue que par certaines de ses localisations, celles qui ont pour siège la gorge et le larynx.

12. Jules Simon, *Nouvelles études sur la diphtérie* (Paris: G. Masson, 1889), p. 8 ; La diphtérie a son bacille spécifique; toute fausse membrane qui contient ce microorganisme est diphtéritique, toute fausse membrane qui ne le renferme pas n'est pas due à la diphtérie.

13. Léon-Henri Thoinot and E.-Jules Masselin, *Précis de microbie médicale et vétérinaire* (Paris: G. Masson 1889), pp. 380–1.

14. Ibid, p. 384. 'De tous les milieux solides, celui qui paraît le plus convenable est le sérum peptonisé de boeuf, de mouton ou de cheval.'

15. François Rabot, 'Prélude à la sérothérapie,' *Lyon médical*, 77 (1894), pp. 527–43.

16. For interesting reflections on the results obtained by Alexandre Yersin in his excursions out of Paris, see Andrew Mendelsohn, 'The Microscopist of Modern Life,' *Osiris*, 2nd Series, Vol. 18, *Science and the City* (2003), 150–170.

17. Michael Worboys, *Spreading Germs: Disease Theories and Medical Practice in Britain, 1865–1900* (Cambridge: Cambridge University Press, 2000) p. 292.

18. Émile Roux, *La Semaine médicale*, vol. 14 no. 51, September 8, 1894, p. 407.

19. *Le Bulletin médical*, 1894. Opposite p. 1095.

20. Moizard and Perregaux, '231 cas de diphtérie traités par le sérum antidiphtérique' *Le Bulletin médical*, 1095–101.

21. M. Funck, *Manuel de sérothérapie antidiphtérique* (Paris: Carré, 1895), pp. 77–8.

22. Georges Lemière *La Diphtérie et son traitement par la sérumthérapie* (Lille: L. Danel, 1895) p. 35.

23. Rabot, for example, published analyses that divided up the success rate of serotherapy in terms of the presence of different bacteria identified in the bacteriological tests.

24. Eugène Aschkinazi, 'Le Stérésol (vernis antiseptique) et ses applications spécialement dans la diphtérie' (MD thesis, Paris Faculty of Medicine, 1893).

Chapter 6

Branding French Serum

One of the major lessons to be drawn from the philosophy of technology as it has developed over the second half of the twentieth century is that the evolution of technology is not just a question of determining the right or the best solution to a technical problem. There is always a range of technological options available and both historians and philosophers have spent much time examining how technological choices are made. This approach, with its emphasis on the multiplicity of credible options and their disappearance following the moment of choice, exploring the mechanisms for establishing a consensual history that underlines the rationality and inevitability of the chosen option, echoes the interest in scientific controversies that contributed to the foundation of the social studies of science a decade earlier. To provide an example of what we mean, we can consider Weibe Bijker and Trevor Pinch's analysis of the development of the bicycle at the end of the nineteenth century, where different, often opposing interest groups oriented the technological choice between competing models. Those (usually young men) with a passion for racing and the sporting use of the bicycle preferred the rapid but dangerous penny-farthing style (a large front wheel turned directly by the rider who sat above it) while the more leisure-oriented user with an interest in less dangerous pursuits adopted the new 'safety' bicycle. This latter model, which came to dominate the market, had a much lower center of gravity thanks to its chain-link rear-wheel transmission.[1] Nevertheless, Bijker and Pinch argue that what might retrospectively be seen as a logical progression (the adoption of the chain as a way to make the bicycle safer, lowering the center of gravity, while maintaining the bicycle's speed) was in fact the outcome of a conflict over the sense and use of a bicycle at the time the option of the chain became available. The moral of the story is that the 'victory' of the safety bicycle was not inevitable, even though it is now difficult to imagine an alternative pattern of development. The bicycle is a particularly rich terrain for this kind of argument, with a number of cases like the one just mentioned of co-existing models that appealed to different groups of users. While one might argue that the bicycle is exceptional in this sense (although there are other 'classic' examples of this kind of technological choice, like the choice between VHS and BETA standards for videocassettes), the implication of Bijker and Pinch's SCOT (Social Construction of Technology) position is that an equivalent argument can be made for all technological developments. Indeed, it is part of a general stance opposing the determinist logic of technological development as progressing unequivocally through successive steps on an evolutionary path with each step representing the best technological solution to the problem at hand in the limit of the means available. Instead, the 'construction' of modern technology is cast in terms of choices among the possible solutions that are related to socially determined considerations rather than just in terms of a functional logic. These social considerations cover a wide range of factors, such as aesthetic taste, lifestyle choices, but often come down to political positioning, with the question of whose choice for what ends coming more and more to the fore.

It is relatively easy to envisage this kind of argument for certain medical drugs, particularly recent ones. Thus, for example, the choice between the 'patch' and the pill form for the administration of a contraceptive is not an entirely 'technical' medical issue and has much to do with the needs of different users with respect to what they expect and demand from their birth-control device, notably its ease of use.[2] This argument seems clearer in other choices between formulations where the pharmacological differences appear to be even slighter. One very French example is the use of the suppository for delivering certain common medical drugs, like paracetamol; a pharmaceutical form limited to relatively few cultural spaces. In the case of the serum, however, it is hard to imagine an alternative to an injection either into a body cavity or directly into the blood stream.[3] Putting the mode of administration to one side, however, we can consider the presentation and prescription for use of the drug in more general terms. In contrast to today's pharmaceutical products, the presentation of the medical drug in its labeled glass phial was not the fruit of any conscious reflection about how best to market the product and there were no formal guidelines for its use, much less a clinical consensus guided by the invisible hand of the drug's producer or the political powers. Furthermore, the Pasteur Institute never engaged in any positive action aimed at 'selling' the medical drug. The dissemination of the information, as we have seen, was via specialist journals and newspaper reports, and while there were advertisements for syringes and diagnostic tests there were none for the serum itself.[4] As early as January 1895, as we shall see in Chapter 8, the Pasteur Institute benefited from a nationwide communication campaign emanating from the Ministry of the Interior, in which the government invited local officials to obtain serum from the Pasteur Institute in case of need. Nevertheless, this was conceived principally as a rationing measure aimed at the rational distribution of a still rare commodity rather than as the promotion of an officially sanctioned product. Furthermore, there were few doctors who had not already heard about serotherapy for treating diphtheria by 1895. At no point did the government issue instructions about when or how the serum should be used.

Even in the absence of any marketing staff or project, we can still think of the Pasteur Institute itself as a brand name, like the names of its leading personalities, Louis Pasteur and Émile Roux, names that were frequently mobilized on the medical marketplace. The serum quickly became associated if not identified with the Pasteur Institute in France, and more particularly with the figure of Emile Roux as Pasteur's successor, an association that was encouraged in certain respects by the members of the Institute. As we have already seen, the circuits of distribution for the serum also favored contact with the Pasteur Institute, either in person or by telegram.[5] Even though the intention of the legislation was for the serum to be distributed to pharmacies across the country where it could be bought with a doctor's prescription like any other medical drug, this model was not widely put into place.[6] Instead, the serum was mostly stocked in government buildings, where the doctors went to collect it. In many cases the serum had to be paid for, but it still escaped the standard circuit of prescription medicines and could often be obtained free of charge. In this way, the serum avoided direct competition with other 'patent' medicines for this disease, and for all the reasons that I have presented in the foregoing chapters it rapidly established itself as the treatment of choice, notably if the presence of the Löffler-Klebs bacteria had been verified by microbiological analysis.

Indeed, the spread of microbiological competence across France was also tied to the Pasteur Institute. The majority of doctors who sought to integrate microbiological techniques into their practices or simply to stay abreast of current developments in the field came to Paris to follow the course in 'microbie' at the rue Dutot. This course was originally taught by Emile Roux, but the teaching was increasingly dispensed by Louis Martin once he was taken on at the Institute. Following the announcement of the success of serotherapy, doctors came to attend the course in much greater numbers, and Martin prepared additional short courses specifically around diphtheria—its diagnosis and treatment by serotherapy—to cope with the increasing demand. In addition, the Pasteur Institute itself provided diagnostic services. These related services provided by the Pasteur Institute can also be interpreted as a form of promotion for the serotherapy, although they were clearly not undertaken with this goal in mind. While they all contributed to the identification of the serotherapy with the Pasteur Institute in Paris, this should not blind us to the fact that the Institute was not the sole producer of serum in France, a subject we will return to in detail in Chapter 8.

THE CHOICE OF AN ANIMAL

One point concerning the production where there seems to have been room for maneuvre was in the choice of animal used to manufacture the serum. In principle, one could imagine a more distributive system, using dogs rather than horses, for example, to produce the serum, although the relatively small volumes of blood one could take from animals this small would have rendered mass production much more complicated. Nevertheless, sheep and goats had been used for many of the initial studies in Germany and in France, and could have continued to be used for manufacturing the serum. For the production of anti-tetanus serum, the Germans experimented with using the milk from immunized cows, aiming at a simplified mode of administration for small children. Although it is difficult to evaluate the functioning of these alternatives that were never put into place, it is important to remember that the horse was a culturally very significant choice in late nineteenth-century France.[7] While horses were to be found everywhere at this time, new technologies were being introduced that would eliminate them from the city and then the countryside. This being said, in a city like Paris there were horses that pulled the trams and delivered goods throughout the city. The army and the police had hundreds of horses at their disposal and almost every farm in the country had its workhorses.

While most of the horses used at Garches to produce serum had been invalided out of the army or were former workhorses from the Paris area, this was not the case for all of them. The use of a public subscription to pay for serum production had some unexpected consequences for the Pasteur Institute's 'cavalry.' Well-heeled donors not only gave money, as will be discussed in more detail in the next chapter, but also horses. As journalists liked to note, at the Pasteur Institute's stables retired thoroughbreds were living side by side with 'common' working horses.

> M. Gaston Dreyfus, the well known sporting man, has proposed for the same service [the serotherapy service] a pure-blood horse, *Salifou*, who has appeared with great success on several race tracks. It is the first time that a thoroughbred has entered the stables of the Pasteur Institute.[8]

These generous gifts served the Pasteur Institute's purposes well, offering an image of Republican equality that mirrored the list of subscribers, open to all; great and small.

The ubiquity of horses not only made their supply relatively straightforward, it also made it easier to find people trained in their upkeep. The staff at Garches had considerably more trouble keeping their stocks of guinea pigs in good health than their horses, because there was no shortage of experienced stable boys, while few people had any practical knowledge of guinea pigs. Today, of course, there are considerably more guinea pigs in the Paris region than horses, but that was not the case in 1895. Having said this, however, this period marks the beginning of the end of the massive presence of the horse in the modern city. First, the bicycle and then the automobile would replace it as the favored means of transport for both human and freight. The irony of this new vocation for the horse was not lost on Gaston Calmette, the journalist for *Le Figaro* who covered serotherapy for the paper, who remarked that producing serum was 'the new mission for horses at the end of the century when the bicycle has sought to dethrone them!'[9] This irony was only heightened by the fact that Emile Roux himself was a keen cyclist. While this reflection on the choice of the horse is interesting, however, I would not want to place a great deal of weight on this argument, but just want to underline how strongly the serum was associated with the horse.

SERUM AND THE FASHIONING OF THE MODERN DOCTOR

The question of how technological objects transform their users is one of the key elements in the development of post-war philosophy of technology. It represents an extension beyond the basic political arguments against the neutrality of technology. If you believe that such objects serve the needs of humans, providing solutions to a variety of practical problems, you might imagine that their use has in return no effect on the user. This logic takes us back to the image of the classic machine, the lever or the pulley, that multiplies human force. In return for the extra capacity afforded by the pulley one is required to pull a rope further than if it were simply attached to the weight to be moved. It is not obvious that using a pulley in this way in turn transforms a person's physical or mental being, or when the practice is generalized, the functioning of a society, let alone people's behavior or attitudes. Nevertheless, the argument that technologies transform not only our lives but also the way we conceive the world has now become a commonplace. There are now many analyses of how technological objects have transformed society at the level of people's mentalities; these analyses originally concerned means of transport, notably the car, the airplane and the space rocket, and more recently information technologies, in particular the computer[10] and communication technologies.[11]

We do not have to search very far to find general arguments about how modern medicine has transformed our relation to our own body, and the functioning of society. In these often critical analyses, medical drugs are generally called upon to play a supporting role, with an idea that pharmaceutical industry pushes unnecessary and excessive drugs on a population of consumers.[12] A number of researchers have argued, for example, that Prozac was not just a novel treatment for depression, but expanded the bounds of the disease, with new definitions pushing formerly healthy people into the category of depressives.[13] Similarly, although in a different domain, Viagra has affected attitudes to male sexuality. In this case, it would be easy to explore how Viagra—presented as a pharmaceutical treatment to help with erectile dysfunction—has transformed its users and the very notion of male sexuality, starting with the generalization of the very term erectile dysfunction understood as a medical condition.[14] This being said, there are a whole range of medical drugs where it is more difficult to see how they could have transformed the patient population (or potential patient population) in comparable ways.

What about serum? We have already seen how bacterial diagnosis redefined diphtheria, allowing doctors to distinguish between those liable to benefit from serotherapy and those not. One could argue that the serum pushed a cohort of otherwise healthy patients into the category of the treatable, particularly if one thinks of the widely practiced but poorly documented prophylactic use as a sort of 'vaccination.' But this is not comparable to the expansion of the category of depression brought about by Lilly's marketing of Prozac. Practices of isolation that were common before the introduction of serotherapy effectively treated the healthy as sick based on empirical knowledge of the infectious nature of diphtheria.

The serum did transform the diphtheria patients in a quite superficial sense, by making them subject to injections of serum rather than the various treatments that existed in the previous decades. Nevertheless, I believe that the most striking transformation brought about by the serum was not of the patients but rather of the doctors who used the new treatment. Consider the outpouring of Paul Persy, a rural doctor who practiced near *Le Mans*. Overwhelmed by the experience, Persy reported his first use of serotherapy in extenso. Here is an excerpt from his rambling narrative:

> On Saturday the nineteenth of January 1895, at around five o'clock in the evening, a farmer from the *Le Mans* region entered my surgery saying: 'I have come, sir, in order to beg you to examine a child with a sore throat as soon as possible' and, he added, now in tears 'you see we are very worried; we lost one to croup four days ago, we only have this one left and "he is going the same way as the first": and we do believe it is the same illness'
>
> 'The child that you lost, was he treated by the new method, was he vaccinated?' I asked
>
> 'No, Sir, we were unable to do so.'
>
> 'Aha!' I said, 'do not despair,

> I am going to pass by the Prefecture on my way and ask for the vaccine and, if it is as you think, and we are dealing with the same disease, you have every reason to hope that your child will be cured.'
>
> 'We would be most grateful, sir, as it would be hard indeed to lose two children in the same week.'
>
> 'It is not me, my friend, to whom you owe your gratitude, but to doctor Roux who found this remedy, and to his master, and a master to us all, M. Pasteur.'[15]

There are a number of lessons that can be drawn from this dramatic story. First, this is a concrete example of the particularly tragic nature of diphtheria. Because it both killed young children and was highly contagious, it could easily kill several children in the same family in a relatively short space of time. The farmer who had already lost one child to diphtheria comes to see Dr. Persy because his only remaining son is gravely ill (we do not know whether he sought out a doctor when the first one fell ill). Dr. Persy is now able to intervene with a new treatment in which he has complete faith. That he can utter the nostrum 'do not despair' with sincerity is vital in the relationship between the doctor and the patient's family. This transformation brought about by the serum was multiplied in hospitals and private practices across France. In return, the doctors' faith in the efficacy of the serum made them de facto advocates for a whole range of associated ideas that we have been considering here, from the germ theory of disease to the value of the government's distribution of a 'national' product provided by the Pasteur Institute. Indeed, Persy's medical adventure required a trip to the prefecture rather than a visit to the pharmacy or simply his own manipulation of the patient. The prefecture adds an implicit official sanction to the treatment that is not without its significance. Persy concludes his account with an ode to Louis Pasteur and Emile Roux.

> Oh Pasteur, Oh Roux, oh beneficent genii! You have conscientiously revolutionized the field of science, and, thanks to your arduous efforts, a superb harvest of blond heads. Ah! That your last hour might be distant and that no suffering—however slight it may be—come trouble the peace of your lives. This is the wish of all those who have the joy and honour to be your contemporaries.[16]

Putting aside the irony that Pasteur would die that very year, we can see in this poem how the doctor represents the diphtheria serum to himself. For him it is both personal and patriotic. The serum is a symbol of the Pasteur Institute, and yet is also a self-representation for French doctors. Those who embraced serotherapy saw themselves as pioneers of a new era in medicine, with diphtheria the first in a long list of successes. Nevertheless, not all doctors shared this view of modern medicine, of the Pasteur Institute or of the anti-diphtheria serum.

RESISTANCE TO THE SERUM

It is very rare to encounter the objections to serotherapy in the historical literature, but it would be wrong to think that everyone was immediately won over by this modern treatment emanating from the Pasteur Institute. Here, it is worth sparing a thought for perhaps the most important actor in the story of serotherapy; the patient, or, in the case of very small children, the patient's family. Recent history of medicine has worked very hard to bring the patient back into the picture, if not to place the patient in the foreground.[17] As with any such history 'from below' the historian is confronted in this case by a problem of sources. The question of the attitude of the patients and their families to serotherapy is evidently interesting and of capital importance but impossible to evaluate. Nevertheless, we should neither imagine that parents were all enthusiastic about this new treatment nor that there was any organized resistance to serotherapy. In reading articles and reports from hospitals one does come across cases (often reported indirectly) where parents refused to have their child treated with the serum. This phenomenon is impossible to quantify, but is certainly very rarely reported and given the relations of authority that operated in French hospitals at the time it was likely to be rare. When the head doctor imposed a form of treatment on a ward, the only way to avoid it was to ensure that one's child did not arrive at the ward. In this same vein, the most likely form of refusal of this treatment (and all the other alternatives discussed at the end of Chapter 5) was simply not to consult a doctor at all.

Putting the patients to one side once again, we can note that not all the doctors were on Roux's side, and many opposed the serum or at least pointed out the dangers associated with serotherapy. While I have not come across any publications that condemned the serum out of hand, the three examples I will consider here cast doubts on the safety of the serum in print.

In the national weekly review for practicing clinicians, *La Sémaine médicale*, a Dr. Mercier reported the observations of a certain Dr. Ausset in Lille. It is clear that this doctor is opposed to bacteriology rather than to the serum itself. He therefore targets the serum as part of a more general campaign.

> M. Ausset (of Lille) based on the observations from his service and his private practice has come out against the invasion of bacteriology that seeks to dethrone the clinic, when the latter should be the only guide in the practice of serotherapy. The presence of the Loeffler bacillus [alone] is insufficient.
>
> This reticence is inspired by the sometimes terrible accidents signaled by some authors following injection of the serum. The author reports his own personal convincing observation. It concerns a child with a benign angina, which when cultured gave the pure Loeffler [bacillus]. The child received 20 cc of Roux's serum. He recovered and left hospital. He returned 12 days after the date of the injection, with a generalized erythema, albuminuria and extreme

prostration. He died 11 days later, with the same symptoms to which a bronchopneumonia was added at the end.

The author concluded that death was from secondary infection of the lung due to the profound disturbance of the child's organism brought about by the injection of the serum. [18]

Dr. Ausset's principal argument is that doctors should not be seduced by the new microbial fad and should continue to have faith in their clinical judgment rather than the results of microbiological analysis. In the end Dr. Mercier, the author of this article, endorsed the use of the serum, which he qualified as excellent, concluding only that the common practice of using serum as a prophylactic should be discouraged because of the disturbance it can cause to the organism.

> Therefore one should not practice what we call preventive injections; one should base one's treatment above all on the general state of the patient. Although Behring's method is excellent, we need to remember that serum, even normal serum, can cause serious accidents that are not inoffensive for the organism.[19]

In a long article that appeared in the local professional journal for the medical community in Lyon, the *Lyon médical* in 1895 entitled 'The other side of the coin (*Revers de la médaille*): what those opposed to serotherapy are saying' the author, Dr. Zolot-Nisky, adopted a more overtly negative position concerning the treatment.

> Now that serotherapy against diphtheria has propagated with such vertiginous rapidity across all civilized countries, we believe it is worthwhile recalling to our readers all the objections that have so far been formulated against this new method. This is all the more useful in our opinion as the adepts of serotherapy, drunk on the striking triumph of modern theories, disdain—perhaps excessively—these objections and the delicate questions that they raise. Perhaps they have engaged too far along this new and unexplored route and generalise the new facts too much, thereby returning insensibly to the old-style approach of treating the disease rather than the diseased as our masters taught us to do.[20]

As with Dr. Ausset, this skepticism is as much to do with the defense of traditional values as the result of any real doubts concerning the value of the serotherapy.

> Once this drunkenness is passed, will it be the same for serotherapy as for an infinity of other panaceas forgotten almost as soon as they are put forward? Will the same fate befall Behring's discovery as that which befell Koch's?[21]

Both doctors, Zolot-Nisky and Ausset, represent a classic conservative medical stance, resisting novelty in their profession in the name of a superior clinical tradition. The serum stood as a symbol for the new bacteriology, which these men perceived, perhaps rightly, as a threat to the tradition of medical practice and ultimately the independence of physicians. In a sense, the conservative position of these doctors was quite prescient, as they identified better than the bacteriology enthusiasts the transformations this new science promised to bring about in medicine.

We will close with a criticism of serotherapy around a specific case in Paris. This case is of interest because it constitutes a direct attack on serotherapy by medical doctors rather than another denunciation of the encroachment of bacteriology into medicine. Ironically, the criticism was initially offered by Paul Moizard, one of the leading champions of serotherapy. Few doctors published more than Moizard on the success of the new treatment and yet his report of a death that he believed to be due to the serum was the only one to evoke a public response from Emile Roux. Moizard presented the case before the Medical Society of the Paris Hospitals (*Société médicale des hôpitaux de Paris*) in July 1895, and the case was reported widely in the specialist press.

The case involved the death of a 6-year-old girl almost two weeks after receiving an injection of 10 cubic centimeters of serum produced by the Pasteur Institute. The bacteriological test came back negative for diphtheria and no further treatment had been administered. Moizard was convinced that the death was a direct result of the serum, and presented the case to the Medical Society of the Paris Hospitals along with Dr. Bouchard on July 5, 1895. He attributed the death to a negative reaction to the serum and believed it was particularly extreme because the serum had been used in a case of non-diphtheritic angina. Nevertheless, Moizard insisted on how unusual a fatal reaction of this type must have been.

> In fact, our case surely concerns a special and truly exceptional sensitivity of the nervous system to the toxins in the serum. It is an isolated phenomenon and will, I hope remain so.[22]

Based on this case, Moizard suggested that in what he termed ‘doubtful cases’ the serum should not be used before the results of the bacteriological test were known. The *Conseil d’hygiène* disseminated this advise through the pages of various journals, recommending that doctors avoid administering the serum before the bacteriological results were known. As we have already seen, however, this practice was widespread and was encouraged by the majority of doctors treating the disease. The general feeling was that delaying treatment represented the greatest threat to the patients suffering from the disease.

Emile Roux was evidently outraged by this whole affair and must have felt particularly betrayed by Moizard. For Roux, however, there was no room for discussion, the fatality reported by Moizard could not be ascribed to the serum, but had to be due to some complicating factor like the presence of a streptococcal infection and he set about denouncing Moizard in print for his incompetence.[23] It is not, however, the details of this debate that interest me here, although they are very interesting in their own right, including an accusation that Roux exerted pressure on leading specialists in the area to muzzle their criticism. What interests me here is what this episode tells us about the room for maneuvre doctors actually had in their assessment of the safety and efficacy of the serum. Once the vision of the serum as a safe and effective treatment for diphtheria was in place, there was little that could be done to dislodge it. The virulence of Roux's response illustrates two things; first how sensitive he was to accusations that he thought might tarnish the image of the serum, and secondly how closely the serum was associated with his name and with the Pasteur Institute. Moizard made no accusation concerning either Roux or the Institute, with neither the quality of the serum nor its efficacy (in treating 'true' diphtheria) being brought into question. In the next chapter, we will explore how this intimate association between Roux and the serum was put into place and how it contributed significantly to the perception of serum in France, or, to put it in more leading terms, how it contributed to the creation of French serum.

NOTES

1. Trevor Pinch and Wiebe Bijker, 'The Social Construction of Facts and Artifacts: Or How the Sociology of Science and the Sociology of Technology Might Benefit Each Other,' in Wiebe E. Bijker et al. (eds), *The Social Construction of Technological Systems* (Cambridge MA: MIT Press, 1987), 17–50. See also Wiebe E. Bijker, *Of Bicycles, Bakelites, and Bulbs: Toward a Theory of Sociotechnical Change* (Cambridge MA: The MIT Press, 1997).

2. Christian Egarter et al., 'Contraceptive Counselling and Factors Affecting Women's Contraceptive Choices: Results of the CHOICE Study in Austria,' *Reproductive Biomedicine Online*, 24, no.7 (2012), 692–7.

3. Although not practiced at first, intravenous injection of serum was later tried in advanced cases of diphtheria.

4. It was illegal to advertise medical drugs in France, but even a casual look at any specialist or generalist journal or newspaper from the end of the nineteenth century suggests that this law was honored more in its breach than in its observance. Furthermore, advertising medical drugs appears to have been a significant source of revenue for publications as diverse as *Le Figaro* and *La Semaine médicale*.

5. Instructions for the use of the serum held in the archives of the Pasteur Institute give 'SERPASTEUR-PARIS' as the telegraphic address for the serotherapy service. This address was put in place as early as 1895.

6. While the majority of the medical drugs sold by pharmacists were still prepared in his 'officine' a growing minority of 'specialities' (the American term 'patent medicine' comes the closest in meaning to this French term) were prepared in bulk by fellow pharmacists who distributed them for sale individually packaged. These products had an unclear legal status and the principal protection the producer benefited from was the brand name or *marque* which could be registered.

7. For an analysis of the importance of the place assumed by the horse in French society, see Daniel Roche, *La culture équestre occidentale, XVIe-XIXe siècle: l'ombre du cheval* (Paris: Fayard, 2008).

8. *Le Figaro* (October 29, 1894), p. 2: 'M. Gaston Dreyfus, le sportman bien connu, nous offre, pour le même service, un cheval pur sang, *Salifou*, qui a paru avec succès dans plusieurs hippodromes. C'est la première fois, croyons-nous, qu'un pur sang entre dans les écuries de l'Institut Pasteur.'

9. Gaston Calmette, 'Le vaccin du croup' *Figaro Illustré*, 2 56 (November 1894), p. 42 'Telle est la mission nouvelle des chevaux, en cette fin de siècle où la bicyclette cherchait à les détrôner!' To this he added the following uplifting commentary: 'Et ne plaignez même pas ces inconscients sauveteurs! Leur jugulaire se referme sans souffrances, à peine ouverte, paraît-il ; puis, dès le lendemain, ils se rapprochent avec la même joie de leur mangeoir encombrée, insouciants de leur destinée, ignorants de leurs bienfaits!'

10. See, for example, the work of Sherry Turkle, e.g. Sherry Turkle and Seymour Papert, 'Epistemological Pluralism: Styles and Voices within the Computer Culture,' *Signs*, 16, no.1 (1990), 128–57.

11. James Everett Katz, *Machines That Become Us: The Social Context of Personal Communication Technology* (Transaction Publishers, 2003)

12. The classic critical text remains Ivan Illich, *Medical Nemesis: The Expropriation of Health* (New York: Pantheon Books, 1976). While drugs feature as part of what Illich terms 'medicalization,' the target of his critique is their overconsumption rather than the drugs in themselves.

13. Paula Gardner, 'Distorted Packaging: Marketing Depression as Illness, Drugs as Cure,' *Journal of Medical Humanities*, 24, 1–2 (2003), 105–30.

14. See, for example, Tiina Vares and Virginia Braun, 'Spreading the Word, but What Word Is That? Viagra and Male Sexuality in Popular Culture,' *Sexualities*, 9 (2006), 315–32 or Jennifer R. Fishman 'Making Viagra: From impotence to erectile dysfunction' in Andrea Tone and Elizabeth Siegel Watkins (eds), *Medicating Modern America*, (New York: New York University Press, 2007) pp. 229–52.

15. Paul Persy, *Ma première application du sérum antidiphtérique*. (Le Mans: Monnoyer, 1895).

16. Ibid, p. 6. 'O Pasteur, O Roux, O génies bienfaisants! Vous avez consciencieusement remué le champ scientifique, et, grâce à vos laborieux efforts, voilà toute une superbe moisson de têtes blondes. Ah ! Que votre dernière heure soit lointaine et que nulle peine, si légère soit-elle, ne vienne troubler la sérénité de votre vie. C'est le voeu de tous ceux qui ont la joie et l'honneur d'être vos contemporains.'

17. Roy Porter reiterated this demand for patient-centered history over thirty years ago, Roy Porter, 'The Patient's View: Doing Medical History from below.' *Theory and Society*, 1985, 14, no.2, pp. 175–98.

18. R. Mercier 'A propos des indications et des accidents de la sérothérapie anti-diphtérique.' *La Semaine médicale*, 1896, p. 396. 'M. Ausset (de Lille), s'appuyant sur les observations recueillies dans son service et dans sa pratique privée, s'élève contre l'invasion de la bactériologie, qui cherche à détrôner la clinique, alors que celle-ci doit toujours être le seul guide pour la pratique de la sérothérapie; la présence du bacille de Loeffler n'est pas suffisante.

Cette réserve lui est inspirée par les accidents parfois terribles que les auteurs ont signalés à la suite des injections de serum. L'auteur rapporte une observation personnelle des plus probantes. Il s'agit d'un enfant atteint d'une angine bénigne, dont la culture donne du Loeffler pur ; cet enfant recut 20 centimètres cube de sérum de Roux. Il guérit et sortit de l'hôpital. Il rentre douze jours après la date de l'injection, avec une éruption érythémateuse généralisée, de l'hyperthermie, de l'albuminurie et une prostration extrême. La mort survint onze jours après, avec les mêmes signes, auxquels était venue, à la fin, se surajouter une bronchopneumonie.'

19. Idem, 'Il convient donc de ne pas pratiquer les injections dites préventives ; il faudra s'inspirer surtout de l'état général du malade ; car si la méthode de Behring est excellente, il faut se souvenir que le sérum, même normal, peut causer des accidents graves auxquels il n'est pas indifférent de soumettre l'organisme.'

20. Zolot-Nisky, 'Revers de la médaille: ce que disent les adversaires de la sérothérapie,' *Lyon médical*, 79 (1895), p. 94.

21. Ibid, p. 94. The reference is to Robert Koch's spectacularly unsuccessful atttempt to introduce tuberculine as a treatment for tuberculosis a decade earlier. For more on this episode, see Christoph Gradmann, *Laboratory Disease: Robert Koch's Medical Bacteriology*. (Baltimore: Johns Hopkins University Press, 2009).

22. Paul Moizard and Bouchard, 'Un cas d'angine non-diphtérique traité par le sérum suivi de mort,' *Bulletins et mémoires de la Société médicale des hôpitaux de Paris*, 12 (1895), p. 530.

23. Émile Roux, 'A Propos d'une observation de MM. Moizard et Bouchard sur un cas d'angine non-diphtérique traité par le sérum et suivi de mort,' *Journal de clinique et de thérapeutique infantiles*, 3, no. 31 (1895), 601.

Chapter 7

Mothers, Children, Serum, Saints, and Scientists

In the preceding chapters, we have been considering the more technical aspects of the production and regulation of serum, as well as looking at its introduction into hospital wards. This approach has had the advantage of allowing us to present the anti-diphtheria serum in depth, and this in a way breaks with the standard vision of the history of medical drugs. The heroic narrative of pharmaceutical progress, particularly pronounced for the period following the introduction of antibiotics in World War II, sees new drugs as the more or less pure products of research whose manufacture and distribution become practically invisible, a natural process following on from scientific innovation. In the present study we have relegated the history of the research around serotherapy to the background in order to concentrate on issues concerning production, an approach that gives a more critical and, I would argue, more profound account of the nature of serotherapy. Nevertheless, the analysis of a medical drug from the point of view of the philosophy of technology reveals the distance between such objects and the machines around which this philosophy has been constructed. The classic image of a machine, like a tractor, a rocket or a rifle, is of an object that can multiply the force of its user, a concept that is difficult to translate into the pharmaceutical arena. So we can once again pose the question with which we started; is it appropriate to consider such objects as technologies? Is the philosophy of technology an appropriate framework for analyzing pharmaceuticals?

Starting from the premise that medical drugs are legitimate examples of technological objects, we propose moving on to examine the serum in domains already touched upon but not sufficiently analyzed in the treatment presented so far. Thus, we will now explicitly open the analysis up to the cultural and political dimensions of diphtheria serotherapy. I will do this in two chapters. The first one covers the more intimate associations or sense of the disease and its treatment—touching on issues of gender and science—while the second enters into much more political considerations, notably the national and international roles of the French serum. I will take this opportunity to present various regional initiatives in serum production that are absent from most historical accounts of serotherapy, even those focusing on France. These production initiatives outside the Paris area, their origins and their fate, tell us something important about the place of serotherapy across the whole of France. Overall, then, the aim of the third and final part of this book is to try to elucidate the cultural and political meaning and function (or rather functions, as they were multiple) of the serum in relation to both diphtheria and France under the Third Republic.

What serotherapy meant to people, both the doctors who administered it and the families whose children were treated with it, built on the deep cultural sense of the disease it was intended to treat. For many of the researchers working on serotherapy, like Roux and Behring, it seemed probable that serotherapy would be introduced first for tetanus, but the anti-tetanus serum was finally made available only after the treatment for diphtheria. While this book has focused on serotherapy for diphtheria, we could equally well have treated the tetanus serum, and the analysis in terms of the more technical aspects of obtaining, packaging and distributing the serum would have been quite similar. Nevertheless, in this chapter we will be focusing on the specificities of diphtheria serum, seeing how both the disease and the treatment fitted into French society and science at the end of the nineteenth century. Thus, we will explore the specific significance of diphtheria as a disease and the influence that this had on serotherapy as a medical drug.

We will start by expanding on the issue of gender that has already been raised in the context of the material conditions of serum production. We use this theme of gender to tie in a second issue that was important in fashioning the image of serum in France; charity—in particular the image of the Pasteur Institute as a charitable establishment modeled on a longstanding Christian tradition of good works. Looking more closely at the functioning of the subscription launched by *Le Figaro* in September 1894, we can see the image (and a certain amount of confusion) this created with respect to serotherapy.

First, then, we return to the issue of gender with respect to the serum, a subject that we already raised in the specific context of production in Chapter 2. The gendered division of labor in the manufacturing process is such a striking feature of the surviving photographic record that it would have been difficult to pass over it in silence, but gender and gender roles contributed to the sense of the serum in a wider sense, reflecting how they informed the disease the serum was intended to treat. Women were very present in the public representation of serotherapy, but this was not because they were expected either to procure or to administer the treatment.

The first woman to receive a medical degree from the Paris faculty of medicine was Elisabeth Garrett in 1870, and the first to qualify as a doctor in France, Madeleine Brès (née Gebelin) in 1875. Thus, at the time of the introduction of serum, while women doctors were just beginning to qualify in small but significant numbers, their use of the serum was marginal. Furthermore, in the increasingly secular world of hospital medicine, male doctors sought to impose their authority over the women drawn from various religious orders who constituted a slowly diminishing majority of their staff.[1] This meant that any innovative treatment like serotherapy was exclusively reserved for the formally qualified medical staff, the doctors and interns. Indeed, the control over such novel, scientific treatments was one of the means for advancing the doctor's interests, particularly in the hospital. Nevertheless, despite the strong hold that men had on clinical practice inside and outside hospitals, certain diseases, notably diphtheria and whooping cough were strongly associated with women. This was neither because women suffered from these diseases more often than men nor because of a higher mortality rate among women and girls, but because they were childhood diseases and at this time children were considered the exclusive domain of women. This vision of a natural (for many, biologically based) division of gender roles, with children being exclusively the affair of women is still predominant in France over a century later. At the end of the nineteenth century, gender divided the French population even more clearly in terms of both their occupations and preoccupations, including their relationship to children. Although anyone could contract diphtheria, and many adults died from it every year, the disease was perceived and represented as a childhood disease, with a much higher rate of mortality among newborns and young children than in the adult population. This perception made the disease of particular concern to women in their role as mothers, a relationship that was emphasized and mobilized throughout the history of the serum.

Serum effectively entered into this relationship. As a new technology, it altered the relationship between men and women around diphtheria on several levels. In the previous chapter we described the change in attitude of the doctors when armed with this new weapon against a particularly deadly disease. Thus, the serum not only benefited from the prestige of the Pasteur Institute and the innovative scientific aura of bacteriology, but it was also injected, a relatively uncommon pharmaceutical operation, adding to the mastery and aura of the doctor. The elaborate routine of preparing the patient and the syringe set the scene for an active intervention that was quite novel to the families looking on. This contrasts sharply with the general feeling of impotence when faced with this deadly disease in the preceding decades, although it would be an overstatement to say that the doctor had nothing to propose for diphtheria victims before the introduction of the serum, as we saw in Chapter 5.

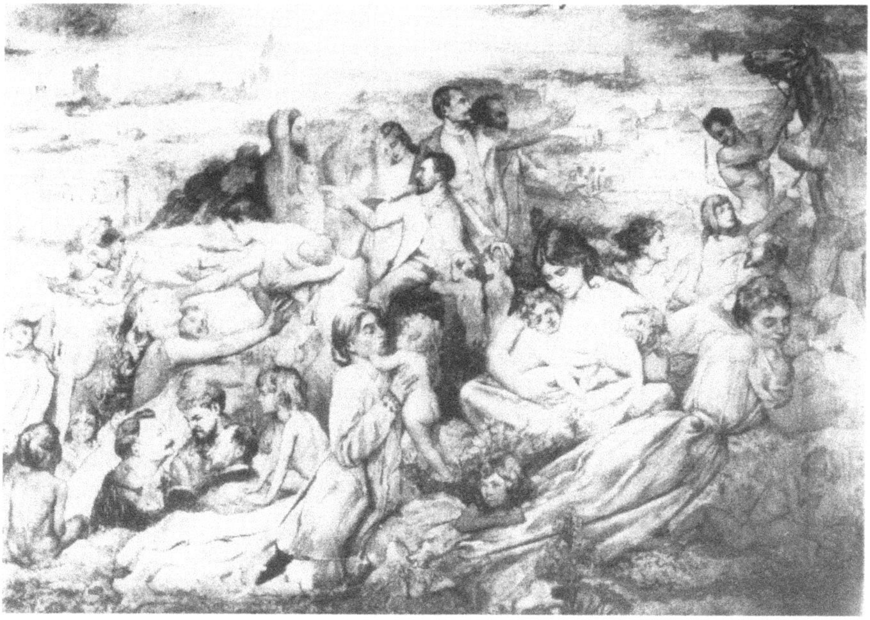

Figure 7.1 ***La sérothérapie*****. Allegory of serotherapy by Charles Maurin (1856–1914) featuring portraits of Emil von Behring and Emile Roux**. Oil painting. *Musée des hospices civils de Lyon.*

The Pasteur Institute, and Emile Roux in particular, occupied a central place in the imaginary of the French serum and this imaginary was strongly informed by images of maternity. In 1895, the symbolist painter Charles Maurin composed a large oil painting entitled 'serotherapy' that celebrated the new treatment. The choice of subject might appear strange for an artist specialized in romantic domestic scenes of mothers and daughters. Nevertheless, as I have just explained, the connection between diphtheria and motherhood was quite evident in the nineteenth century and so the subject of the painting was not as bizarre as it might first appear. Emile Roux is seated right at the center of this large canvas surrounded by contented mothers with their babies and young children. Other researchers like Emil Behring are shown on the margins along with a horse, the provider of the serum.

Whatever the artistic qualities of the painting, it has the merit of conveying several messages quite clearly. First, Roux, his left hand resting on a young boy's head and his right hand pointing at a baby's heart, is the life-giving hero at the center of the scene. Second, the reward for Roux's serum is the boundless maternal love that fills the foreground. This maternal love—given without expecting anything in return—is the model for Christian charity, a principle of loving generosity that would be translated into renewed financial security for the Pasteur Institute. As we will see at the end of this chapter, the corollary of this construction was for the Pasteur Institute itself to be perceived as a quasi-religious institution and its members—Roux first among them—as iconic figures. This understanding of the Institute in relation to the serum added another layer to this particular medical drug as a technological object. It is clear, however, that these considerations and the particular sense they gave to the anti-diphtheria serum apply specifically to the French situation, with the dominant Catholic culture exercising a strong influence on the imagery that was chosen to represent this special relationship. Furthermore, the very financing of the serum production at the Pasteur Institute followed this model, based as it was on charitable donations.

FINANCING SERUM THROUGH CHARITY

While in Germany the serum was produced and marketed by commercial companies, and could be bought in pharmacies like any other pharmaceutical product, this was not the case in France, at least not in the early months of national production. As we have already seen, alternative circuits established themselves and dominated the distribution of the serum in France, with the Prefects intervening directly and privileging hospitals and the network of local health clinics (the *bureaux de bienfaisance*) that had recently been established across France. Roux's intention had been to follow the 'classic' commercial model that prevailed in Germany and Italy—albeit with an ambition to establish a strict monopoly over serum production. For various reasons the manufacture and distribution of anti-diphtheria serum would end up functioning quite differently, occupying a space to one side of the traditional circuit for drugs. Between September 1894 and January 1895 due to the dearth of French serum, the Pasteur Institute limited the distribution of the precious drug to its own network of Parisian hospitals, as well as issuing phials to individual doctors who made the journey to Roux's laboratory on rue Dutot. While the Institute possesses no formal accounts for this period, it is likely that no money was charged for this serum, except indirectly in the ways we will describe shortly. Nevertheless, from the beginning, the Pasteur Institute announced that it would charge for the serum—3 francs per 20 cubic-centimeter phial (the same price as the microbiological diagnostic test presented in Chapter 5)—and that the product would eventually be available for sale in pharmacies (following the obligatory prescription signed by a qualified doctor) like any other prescription drug. There was to be an exception to this policy, planned right from the beginning, for those who could not afford to pay. Poor families could receive the serum free of charge, although this arrangement was subject to payment by local authorities (such as the city of Paris) to cover the cost of production. Although in principle the idea was for the pharmacies to distribute the free phials of serum as well, this never happened and the responsibility for dealing with those who could not pay fell to hospitals, prefectures and the government health clinics. While the Pasteur Institute never hid or denied its plan to sell the serum, it never actively promoted this aspect of its serotherapy program either. To understand why this was the case, we need to look more closely at how the Institute's serum production was funded, a model of financing which explains in large part why the Institute could not in the end function in the same way as the pharmaceutical companies producing serum in Germany.

We have already noted the significance assumed by the announcement made by Roux in Budapest at the beginning of September 1894 in the history of serotherapy in France (as well as the rest of Europe). The journalist (and brother of a researcher at the Pasteur Institute) Gaston Calmette reported this presentation in Budapest for *Le Figaro* using a typically emotive style. The article explicitly addressed the paper's female readership, playing on the tragic links between maternity and diphtheria established across the nineteenth century. Mothers all around the world should, according to Calmette, be grateful to the men of the Pasteur Institute. At the end of his first article from September 6, Calmette appealed in general terms to the French population to support the work of the Pasteur Institute. This casual demand was directed primarily at the government but open to any potential donors, with the vaguely defined goal of improving the handling of diphtheria and possibly building a hospital for infectious diseases attached to the Pasteur Institute. In the days that followed, this quite general appeal for support transformed into a subscription specifically to pay for the production of diphtheria serum and its free distribution to the poor. The subscription was officially launched by *Le Figaro* on September 20, 1894 with a target initially fixed at thirty thousand francs. By the second of October, however, the paper had already received pledges worth 127, 302 francs. The subscription thus successfully combined the virtues of the Third Republic and its model scientific institution with the pathos of diphtheria. The paper published lists of subscribers on a daily basis, with the names of prominent citizens and their large donations sitting side by side with those of provincial schools whose classes had raised a few francs to help combat diphtheria. On October 3, for example, *Le Figaro* published a list featuring M. Léopold Goldschmidt who had pledged 1000 francs as well as 'George V, 3 years old,' who had contributed only three (the cost of one 20 cc dose of the serum). The subscription ended up financing the purchase of horses, and the costly renovation of the Garches site to prepare it for almost a century of serum production. Most of the remaining money was invested, bringing in a regular income to the Institute.

Understandably, the use of a very successful public subscription to fund serum production created a certain amount of confusion among the French population when the serum was eventually put on sale. A letter from February 1895, written by an anonymous donor to Emile Duclaux in his capacity as director of the Pasteur Institute,[2] expresses this confusion, if not outright disapproval in the following terms:

> Is the announcement in the papers correct, that on the tenth of February the Pasteur Institute will be selling serum to the pharmacists? Let me ask you on what you have spent the millions of francs that we have given you?[3]

In his reply, Duclaux argued that there had been a misunderstanding, and presented some doubtful statistics to show that the Pasteur Institute needed the revenues from the sale of the serum to cover its production costs. Nevertheless, the very large sum of money collected by *Le Figaro* was more than enough to pay for the production of serum for several years.[4]

In addition, there was a more specific confusion linked to the serum being made available free to those unable to pay. Although never explicitly stated, the implicit idea on the side of the Pasteur Institute was that local authorities would cover this cost through specific grants to the Institute's serotherapy service. Thus, for example, the city of Paris voted a payment of 15000 francs for the supply of serum in November and December 1894, a payment that was renewed for each of the next two years.[5] Once again, therefore, it is understandable that administrators outside Paris could confuse donations to the subscription with money paid in lieu of serum for their indigent population. Thus, for example, a finance officer from the town of La Motte-Servolex in the Savoie sent 30 Francs to the Pasteur Institute at the end of 1895, which he described as the 'subscription of the Commune of La Motte-Servolex (Savoie) for the purchase of serum.'[6] This phrasing suggests that at least some of those who contributed to *Le Figaro*'s subscription were under the impression that they were buying serum for their local communities, not simply donating money to the Pasteur Institute.

While donors may have misunderstood the nature of the subscription, this was not because they were actively misled; the subscription was a charitable initiative that adopted the model of other such fund-raising projects for epidemics or natural disasters. Nevertheless, it cannot be said that either *Le Figaro* or the Pasteur Institute went to any great lengths to clarify the functioning and status of these various forms of funding. Indeed, the somewhat confused situation suited all those concerned, particularly at the beginning of serum production when it was not clear exactly how the production and use of the product would work out in practice. One reason that a number of people might have assumed that the serum would not be sold but be given to the public free of charge was the model of treatment on which the Pasteur Institute itself had been based. The Institute was set up to provide the innovative vaccination against rabies developed by Louis Pasteur free of charge, and it was against this background that Emile Roux was attempting to impose an appropriate mode of functioning for the anti-diphtheria serum. Looking back to the 1880s and the introduction of the rabies treatment, we can see a number of parallels with serotherapy, which help to better understand the situation of serum in France.

PASTEUR'S HERITAGE AND THE PLACE OF THE PASTEUR INSTITUTE

Even before he founded the institute that would come to bear his name, Louis Pasteur had succeeded in establishing a strong association between the potential of microbiological medicine and children. The first two—widely publicized—official treatments against rabies conducted in Pasteur's makeshift laboratory at the *Ecole Normale Supérieure* saved the lives of two boys, Joseph Meister, 9 years old, and Jean-Baptiste Jupille, 15 years old.[7] Illustrated journals circulated images of this first use of the new rabies vaccine, underlining the hope that an aging Pasteur was bringing to a new generation. Rabies was not, however, considered a childhood disease like diphtheria or whooping cough, and relatively few of those who received the vaccine therapy were children. And yet, these two boys, Meister and Jupille remain enduring icons of Pasteur's rabies treatment, featured in commemorative friezes and statues alike.

The story of Joseph Meister is also highly politically charged. Born in 1876, the young boy lived in Steige, a village nestled in the foothills of the Vosges, between Strasbourg and Colmar, the heart of the Alsace. In July 1885, he was grievously bitten by a dog from the neighboring village of Meissengott (now called Maisonsgoutte). While the story is often told of Pasteur saving the life of an unfortunate French boy, in the terms of the Treaty of Frankfurt signed in 1871,[8] he was in fact saving the life of an unfortunate German boy, or at least a boy from Germany, in a context where the majority of the French, Pasteur included, believed that Alsace should have been part of France.

We will have more to say about the importance of the defeat by the Prussians in the war of 1870 for Emile Roux and the Pasteur Institute in the next chapter when we treat the political connotations of serotherapy in France. Joseph Meister's mother, Marie-Angélique, played an important role in obtaining the experimental vaccine treatment for her son, not only finding Pasteur's laboratory in the rue d'Ulm, but also persuading the reluctant scientist to test his vaccine treatment on her own son.[9] Furthermore, it is not rare to see her represented in traditional Alsatian costume thereby underlining the symbolic role assumed by women with respect to the history of medical microbiology in France, both as mothers and as reminders of wounded national pride.

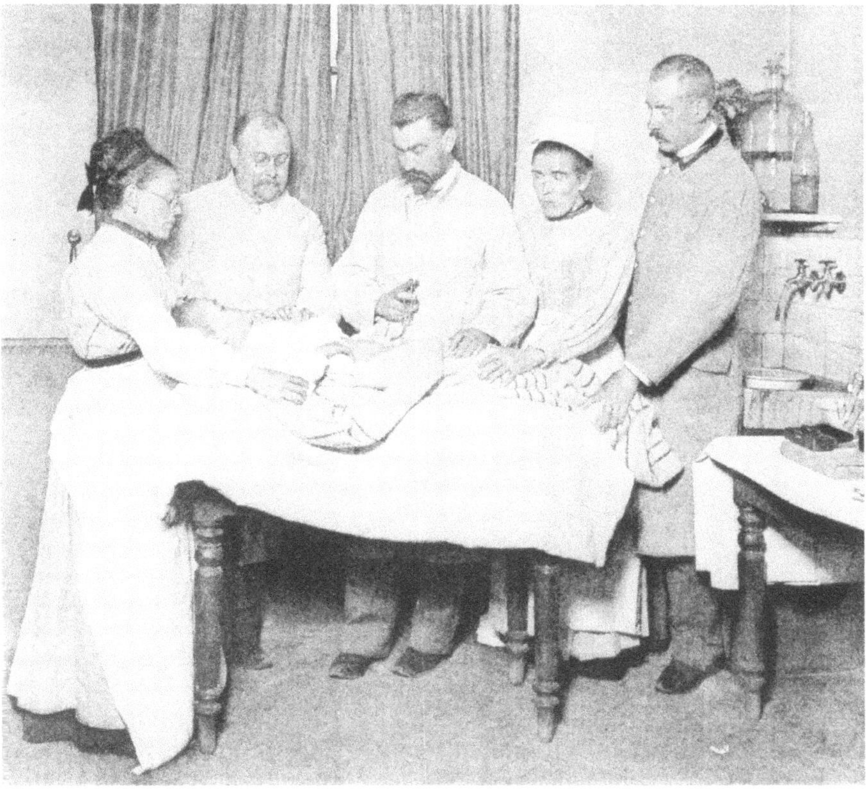

Figure 7.2 Photograph illustrating the administration of the serum at the Hôpital des Enfants-Malades. Figaro Illustré, vol 12, no. 56, November 1894. Private collection, photograph by the author.

In the rich photographic iconography around serotherapy, women feature first and foremost as helping hands in the clinical setting. One of a series of photographs on serotherapy taken for *Le Figaro* in 1894, which we examined earlier when discussing the importance of syringes, shows Auguste Chaillou treating a child at the *Hôpital des Enfants-Malades* helped by four assistants. Two of them are women, Mme Daussoir-Kerleu (or Kerleu-Daussoir, on the left of the picture wearing glasses) and, probably, Mme Gigot, both '*surveillantes*' on the diphtheria ward at the hospital. Like the two male assistants they hold the young boy still while Dr. Chaillou injects the life-saving serum.[10]

The personnel are stiff and the scene is staged in an improvised clinic composed of wooden kitchen tables with sheets thrown over them. The impression given by this photograph contrasts with the atmosphere of a well-known and elaborate oil painting by the medical doctor and artist Georges Chicotot. This picture, painted a decade later, features both a syringe and the anti-diphtheria serum, although they are not at the center of the composition.

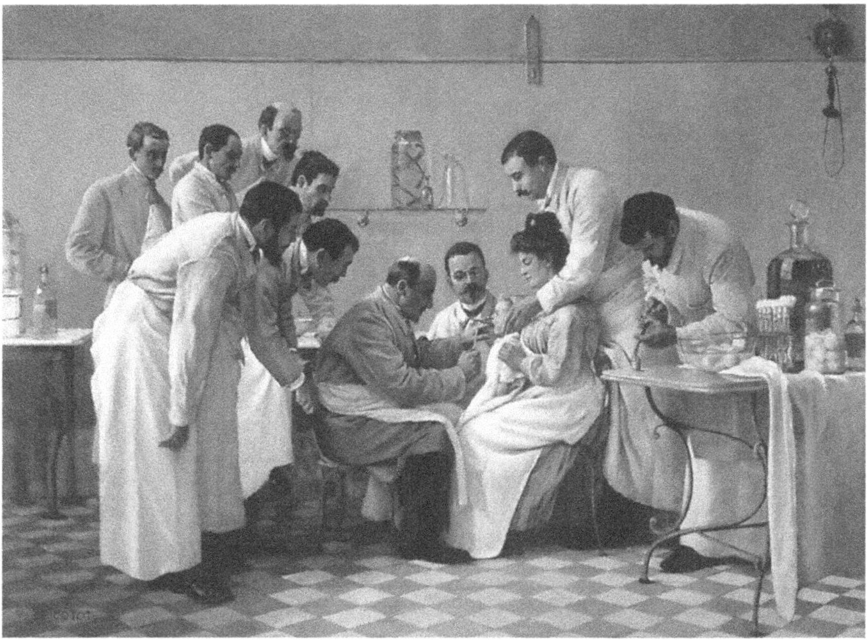

Figure 7.3 Georges Chicotot, Le tubage, oil painting, 1904, Musée de l'Assistance Publique—Hôpitaux de Paris. Photograph, APHP/musée—F. Marin

Furthermore, in Chicotot's painting there is only one woman in a space filled with ten men, and, although probably a nurse, she clearly assumes the situation and the role of a mother. She holds the child by the shoulders and helped by the doctor reaching around her neck to place his hands on the child's head (Dr. Toffemer), we have the impression of the parents holding the baby ready for the expert surgical intervention. While the work is entitled 'Intubation,' and features this surgical technique as its focus, it nevertheless includes serotherapy, with an assistant discretely preparing the injection on the right-hand side of the canvas.

In this painting, Dr. Albert Josias—the director of the pediatric ward at the *Hôpital Bretonnea*u in Paris—is introducing a metal tube through the false membrane of the diphtheria patient to prevent suffocation, the technique of 'intubation' that we discussed at the end of Chapter 5. A radiologist himself, it is perhaps surprising that Chicotot considered this elegant surgical intervention more worthy of his attention than the impending injection, but all but one pair of eyes are on Dr. Josias's manipulation of the intubation equipment. In a way, however, this aesthetic choice serves as a good metaphor for the public representation of today's medicine as much as its perception at the end of the nineteenth century. While medical drugs are called upon to do a great deal of the therapeutic work in contemporary healthcare systems, pills and prescriptions are rarely the subject of documentaries or fiction films featuring doctors, and even less often placed at the center of medical hagiography.[11] There is evidently a philosophical corollary to this phenomenon. When philosophers bring their analytical skills to bear on medical practice it is much more frequently in terms of the definition of health and disease, or the creations of 'cyborgs' via increasingly sophisticated prostheses rather than in terms of the philosophically banal but ubiquitous medical drug.

In a male-dominated world of medicine, diphtheria was a disease that respected the social order. Patients were innocent children, those who cared for them were loving mothers; the only problem in the scenario was that the doctors could not cure the disease. While, as we have seen, this therapeutic impotence is something of a caricature constructed around the perceived success of serotherapy, this vision is nevertheless important in informing the serum as medical drug. With the arrival of serotherapy, the doctor's position, which had hitherto been uncomfortable, was transformed into the preferable stance of effective action. The efficacy of the serum was an extension of a wider efficacy of the treating physician.

The point I want to underline here is that the serum came to occupy a particular cultural space defined in large part by the perception of the disease it was intended to treat. While the serum contributed to forging this space, it did so within a pre-existing context and in relation to various institutions that were also in the process of defining (and, already, redefining) themselves, first and foremost in this case the Pasteur Institute.

In this configuration the image of the serum largely crystallized around the person of Emile Roux, as was clearly emphasized in Maurin's pictoral representation of serotherapy (Figure 7.1). Today, Roux's legend is almost completely eclipsed by that of Pasteur for the reasons that we will lay out in the next chapter. While today Pasteur's shadow obscures all those around him, at the end of the nineteenth century Roux saw himself acclaimed as the new Pasteur. Today, this image of '*bienfaiteur d'humanité*' and the powerful rhetoric of saintly asceticism that surrounded Roux has been largely forgotten, but it was vitally important to the construction of the French anti-diphtheria serum. Roux would eventually assume the direction of the Pasteur Institute, although this institutional recognition of his status took a long time. The evidence for Roux's status as the true heir to Louis Pasteur can be seen most clearly in the Nation's reaction to his death in 1933. The government voted a state funeral for Roux, just as it had for Pasteur, and Parisians came out in hordes to follow his hearse to Notre Dame Cathedral.[12]

The argument here is that in order to understand the serum as a technological object, we need to take into account its situation as a cultural object in France. Much has been written about the ritual aspect of drug use, particularly in anthropology, but here I wanted to underline the importance of cultural

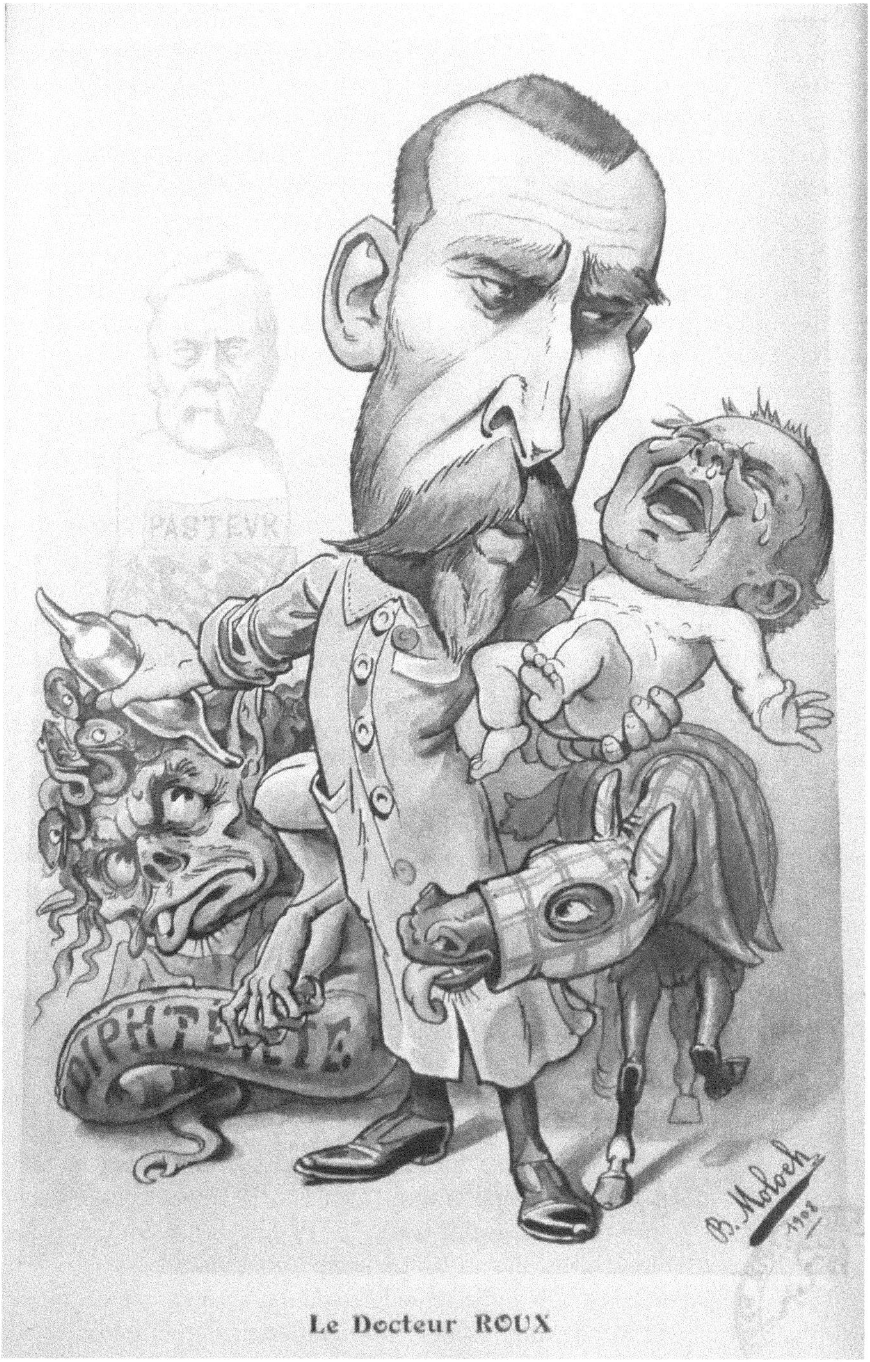

Figure 7.4 Caricature of Emile Roux by Moloch for *Chanteclair*, June 1908. Bibliothèque municipale de Lyon 140 375

associations in shaping medical drugs in specific contexts.[13] Thus, in France, the serum for treating diphtheria was intimately associated with the legacy of Louis Pasteur in the form of the Pasteur Institute, and in particular the figure of Emile Roux.

In this context, the cultural position occupied by the serum also depended on the nature of disease it was used to treat. The serum was a worthy and heroic innovation, bringing protection—represented by the male doctor, in this case Roux—to the family threatened by the disease. Diphtheria was very often illustrated in caricature as a monster, as in this homage to Roux published in 1908 (Figure 7.4).

This illustration brings us to the final aspect of the representation of serum that we will broach in this chapter—its religious connotations. In this caricature published in the bi-monthly promotional magazine *Chanteclair*, Emile Roux is placed in front of a bust of Louis Pasteur. He cradles a crying baby in his left arm; while with a phial of serum in his right hand he holds diphtheria, represented as Medusa, at bay. Roux is looking at the baby with a caring expression and standing underneath the baby we find the faithful horse, the purveyor of the serum. The picture echoes both representations of Saint George and the Nativity scene. The imagery of Roux as the savior could not be clearer. In a biography of Roux by Emile Lagrange, we find a portrait by J.J. Gaillard that represents Roux as Saint Francis of Assisi (loosely based on the painting by Alonzo Cano in Toledo Cathedral), with a list of the diseases he is supposed to have conquered: rabies, anthrax, syphilis and diphtheria. This kind of religious-inspired imagery has been inherited from the time of Louis Pasteur and situates Roux as his successor in the pantheon of secular saints. If medical science was being promoted as the new religion in secular France, Louis Pasteur was its prophet and Roux his leading disciple. The sign of sanctity that Roux holds in his hand is the phial of serum. This treatment against diphtheria was by far the most visible sign of the success of the germ theory. Obtaining and administering this treatment were highly significant acts for doctors and patients alike. It was not just a way to save the life of a small child, but also represented an active participation in a new secular Republic.

Serum can be seen to represent an intermediary object between traditional, conservative, Catholic France and a new secular Republican ideal. While the conservative French tradition promoted family values as well as charity and paternal responsibility, the new Republican ideal transposed a certain number of these virtues onto a secular model, where the citizen was the rightful beneficiary of the care and protection of the representative state. While Pasteur himself embodied a certain conservatism, Emile Roux was of a different political strain, and his choice to defend Dreyfus in the years that followed would doubtless not have pleased his master. In the next chapter we will consider the political connotations of the serum in France in more detail.

NOTES

1. Jan Goldstein explores this tension in her history of psychiatry in nineteenth-century France, see Jan Goldstein, *Console and Classify: The French Psychiatric Profession in the Nineteenth Century* (Chicago: University of Chicago Press, 2001)

2. Duclaux succeeded Louis Pasteur as director of the Pasteur Institute in 1895, when Louis Pasteur became incapacitated by illness.

3. Letter sent to *Le Figaro* for Emile Duclaux, February 1895, *Archives de l'Académie des Sciences*, Paris. Emphasis in the original.

4. According to accounts submitted to the city of Paris, the Pasteur Institute held an investment portfolio of over one and a quarter million francs at the end of 1895.

5. Archives Municipales de Paris, Carton DX6 8.

6. Letter to Emile Duclaux, *Archives de l'Académie des Sciences*, Paris. The problem is a failure to distinguish clearly between '*subvention*' (subsidy), '*subscription*' (subscription), and payment.

7. Whether Pasteur saved their lives is difficult to determine, but the treatments were successful insofar as the two patients survived. They both went on to become employees of the Pasteur Institute, making Pasteur's influence on their lives particularly significant. For more details, including the first experimental treatments using the vaccine that preceded these two cases, see Gerald L. Geison, *The Private Science of Louis Pasteur* (Princeton University Press, 1995).

8. It was this treaty signed on May 10, 1871 between France and Germany in the wake of France's military defeat that officially ceded the Alsace (excluding the territory of Belfort) along with Meurthe and Moselle to the Germans. While the population did not have to become German, those who chose to remain French had to leave the annexed region before October 1872, leading many people to leave the area.

9. In a rare radio interview from 1939, Joseph Meister underlines the role played by his mother. Listen to: 'Vaccin contre la Rage—Interview de Joseph Meister en 1939—TSF' on Youtube (accessed July 22, 2016).

10. The names are given in an article from the same year on an alternative treatment for diphtheria ; Dr. Goubeau and J. Hulot 'Traitement de l'angine diphtéritique par les badigeonnages du fond de la gorge avec une solution concentrée de sublimé dans la glycérine,' *Archives générales de médecine*, 1894, VIIIème série vol. II, 289–418 p. 391.

11. Due to a number of initiatives by historians of medicine, however, pills and prescriptions are now assuming a higher profile in academic histories of medicine. See, for example, the recent collection: Jeremy A Greene and Elizabeth Watkins (eds), *Prescribed: Writing, Filling, Using, and Abusing the Prescription in Modern America* (Baltimore: Johns Hopkins University Press, 2012).

12. See for example, the description of the funeral in *Le Journal* November 11, 1933.

13. See, for example, the edited volume on the consumption of legal and illegal drugs, Jordan Goodman, Paul E. Lovejoy and Andrew Sherratt (eds), *Consuming habits: drugs in history and anthropology*, (London: Routledge, 1995).

Chapter 8

Serum and French Politics

In this final chapter before the conclusion, I will open up the perspective once again to consider the place of both serotherapy and the Pasteur Institute in France at the end of the nineteenth century. Here, I want to look in more detail at the insertion of serum into France's political economy as well as see how different institutions positioned themselves with respect to this medical innovation. Starting with broad reflections concerning the political preoccupations of the last quarter of the nineteenth century in France, I will move on to the more specific aspects of the legislation around serum and how this related to national political concerns about public health issues and how to manage (albeit minimally) the entry of microbiology into medicine. I will then go on to consider a rarely addressed aspect of the history of sera in France, the local initiatives to produce sera in large cities, like Lyon, Marseille and Bordeaux, as well as smaller towns like Le Havre and Grenoble. Examining the cases of Lyon, Grenoble and Nancy, we will see what these local initiatives to produce serum can tell us about the serum, bacteriology, medical education and, more generally, about France under the Third Republic.

This chapter also takes us beyond the serum seen from the perspective of its administration as a treatment by a doctor to a patient in the context of treating a deadly disease. In the following pages we will see how serum served to introduce, or at least to orient, a form of public health initiative around microbiology, first in France and then more specifically in French provincial towns. Indeed, it is intriguing to see how the serum entered into local politics of regional independence if not emancipation from the dominant Parisian institutions. In particular, as we shall see toward the end of the chapter, the local production and supply of serum contributed significantly to medical education across France at the end of the nineteenth century. This being said,

I want to start with the very national or rather nationalistic concerns that helped to shape the perception of serum under the Third Republic in France.

THE DREYFUS AFFAIR AND THE FRANCO-PRUSSIAN WAR

When tracing the excitement around the introduction of serotherapy in the French press, it is striking to see it pushed off the front pages by other breaking headline news of the time such as the death of Czar Alexander III in October 1894 and more particularly the debut of the long-running Dreyfus affair starting in January 1895. This notorious scandal involved the false accusation of spying leveled at Alfred Dreyfus, a Jewish army officer from the Alsace region. The importance that this affair took on, notably when prominent intellectuals like Emile Zola became actively involved in Dreyfus's defense, is impossible to understand without taking into account the background of the Franco-Prussian war of 1870–1871. A quarter of a century after its unexpected humiliation on the battlefield, the French military elite were still searching for an acceptable explanation. While it was unrealistic to expect that they might be able to defeat the German Empire in the foreseeable future, the French were looking for a way to save face, and the idea that a traitor might have given away vital secrets to the enemy was one way of shifting the blame. Although the evidence against him was weak, many, particularly on the political right, were quick to condemn Dreyfus for betraying the Nation, as not only was he Jewish but he also spoke German. Thus, Dreyfus's profile—a Jew from Alsace—made him an ideologically suitable candidate for passing French secrets to the Germans. The anti-German feeling and sense of wounded pride remained close to the surface throughout the 1870s and 1880s and into the 1890s. In particular, the French had never accepted the legitimacy of the annexation of Alsace and Lorraine, and the amputated maps that hung in the offices and classrooms across France served as a constant reminder of this injustice. The French term '*revanchard*' conveys well the paradoxical sentiment that animated France from 1870 until at least 1918, combining the feelings aroused by the recent national humiliation with a keen sense of Republican patriotism. This stance was clearly paradoxical if not straightforwardly contradictory, with the French refusing Prussian occupation and demanding revenge while at the same time searching for the reasons behind their defeat and harboring an unavowable admiration for Germany's advanced modernization program. The Dreyfus affair was symptomatic of this paradox, with the convenient story of betrayal by a Jewish officer convincing enough for many Frenchmen to outweigh mounting evidence of his innocence.

The introduction of serotherapy in France has also to be considered in light of this *revanchard* sentiment that fueled the Dreyfus affair. In the popular press, serotherapy was an example of a success in applied medical science that illustrated how French science, or at least the French scientific spirit, was more than a match for the Germans. The fact that the discovery was seen to emanate from the Pasteur Institute only made this partisan interpretation of the drug more evident. Indeed, the need for such a success doubtless contributed to the attribution of the discovery by certain journalists to Roux rather than to Behring. In his first report from Budapest, Gaston Calmette made the claim quite explicitly.

> It is a French achievement, exclusively French, because, having its origins in the Institute in rue Dutot [the Pasteur Institute], and subsequently tested abroad, it is at this same Institute in rue Dutot that, in the hands of these same men it has been definitively perfected and has achieved its final promotion.[1]

This interpretation of the French origins of the serum also found expression in contemporary 'popular' culture. A local chocolate manufacturer from the South of France provided a set of collector's cards illustrating notable historical events. One such card dealt with serotherapy and featured a picture of the bleeding of a horse adorned with the caption 'Dr Roux, Pasteur's student, discovers the remedy against diphtheria.' While the explanation on the back of the card is more circumspect concerning the relative contributions of French and German scientists to the discovery, it nevertheless concludes by once again foregrounding Roux's contribution.

> Thus we see this barbarian diphtheria—the scourge of children, the terror of mothers—all but defeated thanks to the patient research of Doctor Roux, the tireless student of the Great Pasteur.[2]

The author readily mobilizes a number of clichés, including all the stock references for the diphtheria serum; mothers, Emile Roux and 'the Great Pasteur.' We need to recall, after all, that Louis Pasteur was not only Roux's employer, but also the foremost scientific figure in France's revanchard pantheon. In 1870, his son had enlisted to fight for France, and upon hearing the news of the bombardment of the Academy of Sciences in Paris by the Prussians, Louis Pasteur had publicly returned his honorary doctoral diploma to the Faculty of Medicine in Bonn. This stance and other outspoken criticisms of the conduct of the invading army earned Pasteur an enduring reputation as the embodiment of French national pride under the Third Republic.[3]

In 1871, while he was taking refuge in Lyon, Pasteur published a vituperative article in the *Salut Public* in which he quite clearly expresses his ambivalent feeling toward the Germans. While he was not afraid to express his disdain for the ambitions and strategies of *le chancre prussien* (the Prussian canker), Pasteur nevertheless explained how much he admired the Prussian policy of investing in science that had raised them up to a dominant position in Europe over the preceding fifty years. This dominance was, according to Pasteur, across the board; in industry, research and education, with the German university system establishing itself as a model for the other European nations. Where Germany had succeeded, Pasteur bemoaned, France had failed:

> Here, I propose to demonstrate why at the moment of its supreme peril, France did not find the superior men needed to mobilize the resources and courage of its children. This must be attributed, of this I am convinced, to the fact that France has, over the last half a century, failed to take an interest in the major works of the human mind, particularly the exact sciences.[4]

This logic would lead him to the project for the Pasteur Institute as a site for research and teaching in France, an important step down the path to reconquering the exact sciences for his homeland. Over a decade after the Franco-Prussian war, with his star on the rise, and in particular thanks to the celebrity that accompanied the introduction of his treatment against rabies in 1885, Pasteur was the living proof that French scientists were the equal of their German counterparts. Indeed, as we have already mentioned, the Pasteur Institute was quite literally built on the success of the rabies vaccine, and became an integral element in the post-war discourse around France's revenge on the Germans.[5] It was the *Acadêmie des sciences*—whose bombardment had so outraged Pasteur—that launched the subscription to pay for the new building in 1886. Two years later, after raising funds from around the world, the state organized an inauguration ceremony that made the front pages of newspapers across France. Although in poor physical health, Pasteur insisted on attending the dedication of this building that would perpetuate his scientific memory for centuries to come. His speech, which was read out by his son, once again played on memories of France's defeat and concluded by pointing to the ultimate victory of the French on the higher moral battlefield of the medical sciences.

> [T]wo opposite laws seem to be at war today; a law of blood and death . . . and a law of peace, work and salvation that only aims at delivering man from the scourges that plague him; while one only seeks violent conquest, the other relieves humanity; the latter values a single human life above all victories, the former sacrifices hundreds of thousands to the ambition of one man. . . .
>
> Which of these two laws will win out over the other? God alone knows! But what we can say with certainty is that French science will force itself, in conformity with this law of humanity, to push back the frontiers of life.[6]

While science and technology were making war ever more deadly, the medical sciences held forth the promise of salvation. On the side of the

humanity of modern medical science, Pasteur cites life-saving antiseptics, but he is also thinking of his own treatment against rabies that offered a new scientific response to an otherwise untreatable deadly disease. The subscription that had raised the money for the new building was launched with the explicit aim of providing an independent site where the treatment against the disease would be available to all callers, free of charge. Pasteur endowed the institute with a triple mission which would ensure its future, facilities for providing rabies treatment would be accompanied by research and teaching in the field of microbiology.[7]

The Pasteur Institute became a model as well as a bargaining chip across Europe. Pasteur's German rival Robert Koch quickly put it to use in his attempts to procure his own institute in Berlin. While he worked for the recently founded Imperial Health Office, starting in 1887 he successfully campaigned for a German equivalent of the Pasteur Institute and in 1891 the 'Koch Institute' was founded, attached to the Charité hospital in Berlin. The British also sought to emulate the Pasteur Institute. Meetings of medical dignitaries held in the Egyptian room of the Mansion House Group in London in 1889 aimed to found a Pasteur Institute in Britain.[8] This would be a place not only for patients to receive Pasteur's new treatment against rabies but also for scientists to undertake microbiological research and to disseminate the new microbiological discoveries. In the end, officially for financial reasons, but probably more because of fears associated with anti-vivisection activism (the anti-vivisection act passed in 1876 introduced restrictive licensing requirement for any animal experimentation), the choice was made to use the money to finance voyages to Paris for treatment instead. A number of men continued to lobby for an institute in Britain (either in London or in Cambridge) and two years later the announcement of the new Institute could be made at the Tenth International Congress of Medicine held in London. What would come to be known as the Lister Institute was initially founded as the British Institute for Preventive Medicine (BIPM) with four explicit missions:

1. To study, investigate, discover and improve the means of preventing and curing infective diseases of man and animals.
2. To provide instruction and education in preventive medicine to medical officers of health, medical practitioners, veterinary surgeons and advanced students.
3. To prepare and supply to those requiring them such special protective and curative materials as have already been found or shall in future be found of value in the prevention and treatment of infectious disease.
4. To treat persons suffering with infective diseases or threatened with them, in buildings of the Institute or elsewhere.[9]

Like the Pasteur Institute, the BIPM was privately funded through subscription, and it too manufactured its own serum beginning in 1894. Nevertheless, unlike the Pasteur Institute, the BIPM never established itself as a dominant producer in the UK, as there was considerable competition on the British market both from not-for-profit institutional ventures like the Leicester Bacteriological Institute, and from private companies like Burroughs, Wellcome and Co.[10]

While the serum was not at the origin of microbiology and was not *the* reason for the founding of all these major research institutes across Europe (the Pasteur Institute, the Koch Institute and the Lister Institute), it nevertheless provided an important boost to these projects, and for many of them served as a vital source of income if not, as in the case of the Lister Institute, the impetus behind their foundation. In France, there is a serious doubt whether the Pasteur Institute would have survived for very long had it not received the influx of money from the subscription, subsidies and sales associated with the anti-diphtheria treatment. As Paul Weindling has pointed out, while the Pasteur Institute succeeded in raising large amounts of money for investing in the construction of its building and start-up costs, it got by with little public or charitable finance to pay its staff and other running costs, at least compared to its German rival, the Koch Institute.[11]

So, although serum was not at the origin of this international rivalry around microbiology and its associated institutes, with its wide pharmaceutical potential and its clear message for the importance of microbiology for public health, serotherapy had a major influence in the concretization of and support for such national projects. On October 23, 1894, the president of France paid a visit to the Pasteur Institute. Jean Casimir-Perier had been elected president in June of that year following the assassination of the last president, Sadi Carnot, in Lyon. Presiding over a Conservative government with a rival presidential candidate as prime minister, Casimir-Perier would only last another three months after this visit before resigning and withdrawing from politics. The visit to the Pasteur Institute was in recognition of the importance that serotherapy had already assumed, and Casimir-Perier not only decorated Roux, Martin and Chaillou, but he also went to the *Hôpital Trousseau* to witness the administration of the serum in Paul Moizard's diphtheria ward.[12]

> Before raising Roux to the rank of Commander in the *Légion d'Honneur*, the French President made a short speech.
>
> You have merited this award by all your work and your admirable research on serotherapy as well as by its recent application to the treatment of diphtheria.
>
> Answerable to public opinion, a government is content when it has only to interpret the sentiments of the Nation, and it is in reality the Nation that awards you its gratitude.[13]

Casimir-Perier doubtless saw this visit and his praise for the Pasteur Institute, like serotherapy itself, as a consensual public gesture without any particular risk in what was a tense political situation. In terms of its practical engagement, however, at the time of this visit the government was not assuming any responsibility with respect to the serum, beyond the not insignificant act of subsidizing its production by the Pasteur Institute. As we have already remarked, the Pasteur Institute's serum only became widely available across France in the first months of 1895. By then, the dissemination of large amounts of serum outside the traditional circuit of pharmacies cried out for some kind of official action, or at the very least official recognition of the situation. In case of a major accident, not to have said or done anything would have been inexcusable. Here the history of what had happened in Germany a decade earlier must have exercised a considerable influence on political calculations.

In 1880, Robert Koch had announced the discovery of a treatment for tuberculosis which he called Tuberculine.[14] Desperate patients flocked to Berlin in the hope of a cure. It soon became apparent that the treatment not only did not work but was also probably dangerous in its own right. The unsuccessful, if not to say disastrous, launch of Tuberculine threw a harsh spotlight on the risks posed by unregulated medicines. Although it did not seem to have any lasting consequences beyond generating general skepticism concerning innovative microbiological medicines, the German government was quick to react to the introduction of serum in Germany with stringent regulation. The French too were aware of the risk of the serum turning out to be another Tuberculine episode. More politically damaging than any public outcry about a dangerous drug, however, would have been a public outcry about government negligence.

FRENCH LEGISLATION ON SERUM: THE LAW OF APRIL 1895

Looking in detail at the origin and development of the law of 1895 covering serum helps us both to gauge the significance of the drug to France's elected representatives and to locate the serum within this political sphere. The debates in and out of the National Assembly as well as the legislation that was finally introduced are yet more elements that helped to shape the serum as an object in France. We have already raised this issue when we considered the evaluation and labeling of the product, but looking at the debates around the law gives another, wider perspective as well as providing an opening into the local production initiatives that will be the subject of the closing part of this chapter. The legal status of the serum, as we have already argued on several occasions, was constitutive of the object as it circulated in France.

It influenced not only what was written on the label but also how the object was perceived and used by doctors and patients' families alike.

As we have already remarked, when the serum was introduced in France at the end of 1894, it was covered by no legislation, as it was not officially recognized as a medical drug or as any other particular kind of merchandise. The government's first initiative when confronted with this new product in France was to take advantage of a legislative project on pharmacy already under consideration and introduce a new article that would cover not only serum but also all the various other microbiological products that had appeared on the market at the frontiers of traditional pharmacy.[15] Thus, the government could take advantage of this opportunity to make a clean sweep, bringing some order to this rapidly expanding fringe area of medicine.[16] In the end, article 14 of the draft law on pharmacy from January 1895 proposed the following solution to this group of problems.

> Article 14.—No substances, such as attenuated viruses, therapeutic sera, modified toxins and analogous products that can serve as prophylaxis or therapy for contagious diseases, can be debited either free or against payment until they have received a government authorization, which will be granted following the recommendations of a consultative committee for public hygiene and the academy of medicine.

The approach envisaged by this law was to form the basis of the legislation that would be voted into law three months later. The government (via the Ministry of the Interior) was to allow the sale of these products only after the products themselves had been authorized (provisionally) by the government. The Ministry of the Interior was not planning to take care of these authorizations itself, however, but would devolve this responsibility onto an expert technical committee. Thus, the law called for a special committee working in collaboration with the academy of medicine in Paris to make recommendations to the Ministry. While the Ministry was free to accept or to refuse these recommendations, it was understood that the decisions would essentially be taken by the committee. The article closed by specifying that 'the product will be delivered to the public by pharmacists. Each bottle or recipient will carry the mark of its place of origin and the date of its fabrication.'[17] Article 14 also explicitly extended the pharmacist's monopoly to the distribution of these substances. Nevertheless, while the demand for traceability through labeling, similar to that made of any other mass-produced pharmaceuticals, would survive into the final law on sera, the exclusive right of the pharmacists to sell these products would not.

After having been approved by the Senate at the end of 1894, this draft law failed to pass the next hurdle of approval by the National Assembly.

Meanwhile, the Minister of the Interior, Georges Leygues, decided that the situation concerning serotherapy was too urgent to let the provisions concerning its regulation flounder with the rest of this text aimed at reforming French pharmacy. Thus, he set about salvaging article 14 by detaching it from this faltering pharmacy project. His initial solution was to insert the relevant clauses into a finance law that allocated a subsidy of 80,000 francs to the Pasteur Institute, a 'subsidy' to be made in return for the Institute providing serum to the poor free of charge, the national equivalent of the 15,000 francs already paid by the city of Paris. Although this legislative fix was rejected on technical grounds, it nevertheless imposed a significant change in the prospective law. As serum would be provided free in certain circumstances, the pharmacist was no longer required to participate in its distribution, notably when the serum was deposited at a *bureau de bienfaisance*, the new network of local dispensaries catering to the poor. It was, then, this detour through the finance law that put an end to the project of inserting serum into the standard circuit for the distribution of medicines in France via the pharmacist. This exclusion of serum from the pharmacist's monopoly over medical drugs in France was more than just a coincidence, because, as we have already remarked, the promise to make the serum available for free to indigent patients was bound into the subscription organized by *Le Figaro* in 1894.

Leygues finally resolved the legislative problem by drafting a specific law on serum and associated products, a text that he pushed through the two houses on an emergency schedule. This law was the subject of debate in both the National Assembly and the Senate before being approved and signed into law by President Félix Faure (Casimir-Perier's successor) on April 25, 1895. The text consisted of four articles, with the last two specifying the penalties for contravening the law. While essentially the same, the terms of the first two articles differed in several significant details from the original article 14 of the draft pharmacy law on which it was based. First, its scope was somewhat broader, covering 'Attenuated viruses, therapeutic sera, modified toxins and analogous products that can be used prophylactically or for the treatment of contagious disease, and chemically undefined injectable substances of organic origin. . . .'[18] Furthermore, while the original version envisaged authorizing each product individually, the final law specified that the approval process could be applied to either the product's manufacturer or its origin. This apparently minor change was of particular significance in fashioning serum production in France, as in the end no specific product was ever approved by the Serum Commission, only manufacturers.

Article 2 of the law started by reaffirming the exclusive right of the pharmacists to sell the products only on prescription as well as the need for labeling, measures that were already present in article 14 of the draft pharmacy law, but it then went on to enumerate the exceptions. First, doctors could provide the serum directly to their patients in case of emergency, although how they could obtain the treatment was not specified. Second, in line with the abortive finance text, the product intended for distribution to the poor free of charge no longer needed to pass through a pharmacy. Provided the glass was embossed with the words '*Assistance publique—gratuit*' (Public aid—free of charge), the phials could be delivered directly by the producer to approved sites for subsequent distribution to hospitals and doctors. Although the intention was to provide this serum to those who could not pay, it seems that the result was a much more general circuit of distribution where doctors and patients could obtain the serum free of charge.

The debate over the law in the National Assembly was brief but lively, with opponents and supporters alike caught short by its introduction via an emergency debate and vote. Some elected representatives questioned the urgency of the matter, with several members arguing for the debate to be delayed to give them time to prepare their responses. But the emotionally charged arguments concerning the death of children from diphtheria due to the use of ineffective serum carried the day. Odilon Lannelongue, a doctor and deputy claimed that he had evidence of the existence of clandestine producers distributing dangerously ineffective serum.

> There are secret manufacturers of serum; they make poor quality serum that is dangerous. Do you or do you not want to give them the right to circulate it; that is to the say the right to kill people?[19]

In light of these kinds of emotive arguments, the deputies were under pressure to approve the law as soon as possible or suffer the electoral consequences of having been inactive in the face of an imminent threat to the lives of their constituents' children. The main arguments offered against the content of the law were not nearly as specific, and principally concerned the appropriateness of state intervention in this area. Several deputies argued that the restrictions imposed by the law would interfere with the freedom of research and development, although the logic of this position is not very clear. Following a more lucid line of argument, although full of praise for Pasteur and Roux, the outspoken deputies opposing the law saw it as preparing the way for the state-sanctioned monopoly of the Pasteur Institute over the production of diphtheria serum. Notwithstanding, the deputies were apparently convinced of the urgency of the situation and the very real threat posed by illicit serum production, and the law was approved in the same emergency session by 516 votes to 2.

The government was evidently confident of its victory, because even before this vote, a decree had been circulated restricting the distribution of serum in anticipation of the legislation. Thus, at the beginning of March 1895, the official government journal carried the following note:

> Until the promulgation of the law on pharmacy, one can only deliver serum in France, whether free or against payment, whose fabrication or provenance has been approved by the Ministry of the Interior, following the opinion of the Academy of Medicine and the Consultative Committee on Public Health.[20]

Starting with this decree, but formalized by the president's signature in April, the serum fell squarely under the regime of French law; none could be supplied to patients without official approval of either the product or the producer. It is ironic that this decree was published in anticipation of a law covering pharmacy that was never approved, but, as we have just seen, it was quite appropriate for the text signed into law the following month. The administrative framework was now in place, but there was as yet no advisory committee to the Ministry of the Interior. This panel charged with evaluating the candidates for serum production, known as the Serum Commission, was in turn constituted on May 15, 1895. It was to be composed of sixteen members, half appointed as a direct function of their administrative position, and the other half chosen by the Ministry of the Interior.[21] Out of the eight named by the Ministry of the Interior, four were members of the Academy of Medicine, and the other four drawn from the Consultative Committee for Public Health. The four chosen from among the ordinary members of the Academy of Medicine were Edmond Nocard, Emile Duclaux, Isidore Straus and Jacques-Joseph Grancher, all prominent pastorians, including the director of the Pasteur Institute himself, Emile Duclaux.

What are we to make of this overrepresentation of 'interested' parties from the main serum producer in France on the committee that was charged with providing official approval to such producers? This situation, which by today's standards would be considered an obviously unethical conflict of interest, can be interpreted in at least two ways. Either it was the tacit recognition by the government that the Pasteur Institute was *the* official producer of French serum, or it was a constrained but unintended outcome resulting from the monopoly of the Pasteur Institute over the relevant microbiological expertise. If the Commission was to be charged with inspecting and evaluating potential producers of the serum, its members (at least those assigned these inspection duties) had to possess the relevant knowledge for carrying out these duties. In a context where microbiology was neither studied nor taught in medical faculties or universities in France, the Pasteur Institute was the only source of such expertise. Whatever the reason behind it, the constitution of this committee gave the Pasteur Institute control over the production of anti-diphtheria serum in France, as it thereby held the key to the French authorization process. The outcome that we might expect from this configuration would be an even closer association between the Pasteur Institute and serotherapy, maybe even a monopoly, a wish expressed by Emile Roux himself. In 1894, Roux had publicly argued that only the Pasteur Institute could be trusted to produce safe serum, and letting others do so would represent a risk to public health. Nevertheless, the outcome was not the Institute's monopoly over production, as the Commission approved other regional French producers.

The first list of approved manufacturers of the diphtheria serum was published on January 26, 1896. Unsurprisingly, the Pasteur Institute in Paris appeared at the top of the list followed by the Pasteur Institute in Lille.[22] Four other institutions received approval for the production of diphtheria serum in this same list; serum manufacturers from the towns of Le Havre, Nancy, Lyon and Grenoble.[23] These local institutions were joined by others in towns like Marseille and Bordeaux in subsequent lists of approved centers. While they would never constitute any threat to the Pasteur Institute's dominance in the field, these provincial serum producers are interesting in terms of what they can tell us about the politics of local public health and the perception of serum as a local or national product. Here, I will focus on what regional serum producers contributed to the situation, notably their relationships to public health institutions and medical faculties. Thus, I will argue that the serum was critical in introducing bacteriological teaching into a number of regional medical faculties. This association reinforces an argument I have already made about microbiology being an important element in the sense assumed by the serum in France. From this perspective the detour through the French 'provinces' allows us to see the concrete implications of the introduction of serum in a domain as important as medical education.

SERUM IN THE PROVINCES

The front-page story of Roux's announcement at the international hygiene conference held in Budapest found in *Le Figaro* was reprinted and commented upon across France, with Lyon's *Le Salut Public* publishing their version of the report on September 7, 1894. The newspaper adopted the optimistic picture of the treatment proffered by Roux and disseminated by *Le Figaro*:

> As for its use, nothing could be simpler, with a single injection almost always being sufficient. M. Roux has never given more than two injections to any child with diphtheria. He injects 20 cubic centimeters in one shot under the skin at the side (of the abdomen); straight away the temperature falls, the false membranes

> that suffocate the patient stop growing within twenty-four hours, detach after thirty six, and the bacillus disappears from the throat.[24]

This was probably the first time that the majority of doctors in the Lyon area had heard about serotherapy and it must have appeared to offer a miraculous breakthrough in the treatment of diphtheria. Nevertheless, it seems that the first to be able to use the serum to treat the disease in Lyon only managed to do so a month later. This was François Rabot, the head of the diphtheria ward at the *Charité* hospital, part of Lyon's *Hospices civils*. In December 1894, he recounted his experience with the serum to Lyon's Medical Society, and I will have more to say about this first use of the serum later. Like the wider public, Rabot had been alerted to the existence of the serum by the news reports of Roux's presentation in Budapest in September 1894, and had initially tried to obtain the treatment directly from the Pasteur Institute in Paris. Like practically all the provincial doctors who contacted the Institute, Rabot's request was denied. Coupled with the inflated promotion of the serum, this refusal spawned a sense of bitterness that was probably widespread among specialists (and maybe many generalists as well) outside Paris. This is what Rabot had to say about the experience:

> I cannot say anything about the serum from the Pasteur Institute because I have never had any. I cannot, however, remain silent concerning the curious situation in which provincial doctors find themselves. There is now an infallible remedy for diphtheria, but this remedy can only be used in Paris.[25]

This sentiment of frustration was a key element behind the reactions to serum outside Paris. The print media played a paradoxical role in this story; presenting the treatment as an infallible, almost miraculous cure for diphtheria their exaggerated praise guaranteed immediate demand across the whole country, but the limited supply had the result of converting this thwarted demand into equally widespread frustration. At the Pasteur Institute in Paris, Emile Roux was only too aware of the problem of a limited supply of serum outstripped by a sudden massive demand, but he could do nothing about it because of a logistical problem related to the production of serum in horses. It took a minimum of two months to make a horse ready for serum production by immunizing against successively more potent doses of the diphtheria toxin. With only a handful of horses ready in September 1894, Roux knew that even after he had bought the hundred horses he esteemed necessary for meeting national demand, the serum from the Institute's 'cavalry' would not be available before early in 1895. This is how he recalled the situation in a retrospective report on the serotherapy service he prepared for the director of the Pasteur Institute.

> Requests for serum came from everywhere, and like a rising tide threatened to submerge the bacteriologists. As for us, we would never have believed such a rapid success possible, we thought that like all good things, the serotherapy for diphtheria would only be introduced slowly, and so we only prepared enough horses to supply the hospital services, and our poor animals, even at the cost of giving up all their blood, would not have been capable of furnishing one hundredth of the required quantity.[26]

Roux's immediate response, as we have already seen, was to restrict the distribution of serum, limiting the supply of the precious drug to the Paris hospitals. One consequence of this policy was that those who disposed of the means brought their children to Paris for treatment. At the *Hôpital des Enfants-Malades*, where Roux had first tried the French serum, the hospital staff witnessed a sudden rise in admissions. As this note from the head nurse makes clear, the hospital was ill prepared for this influx of patients.

> I informed M. Gallet that children from the provinces were flocking in to benefit from Dr Roux's treatment, and that we needed to prepare for the diphtheria service to be congested in a very short time. M. Gallet authorised me to open a ward of eight beds under the nursery and to exact payment from those children who could afford it.[27]

Another effect of this lack of serum from the Institute Pasteur was the generalized frustration outside Paris that we have already seen expressed by François Rabot. Dr. Gabriel Roux, the director of the Municipal Office of Hygiene in Lyon had a similar experience when, following the news reports from Budapest, he was asked by the mayor of Lyon (Antoine Gailleton, himself a medical doctor and former Chair of Cutaneous and Syphylitic diseases at the new Faculty of Medicine and Pharmacy in Lyon) to obtain serum for the city. In a report to the mayor, Roux explained the response, or rather lack of response he had received from the Pasteur Institute, and laid out the possible alternatives for the city.

> The Pasteur Institute briefly replied to me that the antitoxic serum would not be sent out to the provinces within the next two months, and then would only be delivered to hospitals and patients signed up with the 'Bureaux de bienfaisance' [28]

Faced with this refusal, Gabriel Roux suggested in the same report that, like its neighbors Saint Etienne and Grenoble, Lyon should make provisions for producing the anti-diphtheria serum itself. This task would be entrusted to Saturnin Arloing, a professor at both the medical and the veterinary schools in Lyon, who already had some experience in research in microbiology. Profiting from the facilities at the two schools and subsidized by the city, Arloing launched the immunization process on a pair of horses.

But Gabriel Roux's ambitions did not end here. He used the interest around the serum to lobby for an extension of the 'bureau d'hygiène' in the center of Lyon. This municipal medical facility was where vaccination and other treatments were made available to the city's population, and it was here that serum would be distributed to the poor. Roux suggested that the services for distributing the serum should be coupled with the on-site capacity for diagnosing diphtheria by examining samples taken from patients under the microscope. This would require constructing a small extension to the existing building in which there would be a room for the diphtheria patients apart from the others (to minimize the risk of infection), and the means for performing bacteriological diagnoses.

Arguing that the facility would not be very expensive (it would be composed of four rooms over a modest 100 square meters), Roux insisted on the need to be able to diagnose diphtheria in order to use the serum effectively.[29] Although Gailleton did not immediately fund this project, following the persistent assertion of Lyon's need for a municipal bacteriological diagnostic laboratory, Roux eventually got his way. In light of the struggle involved in obtaining this laboratory explicitly tied into the introduction of the serum in Lyon, it is hard to imagine that without the serum Roux would ever have succeeded in financing the project. Perhaps one reason that Gailleton did not finance the project straight away was because it did not offer a solution for the local supply of serum, as the project only covered its distribution and the on-site diagnosis of diphtheria. In the end it was Lyon's new Faculty of Medicine that would take care of production, with Saturnin Arloing placed in charge of the project, as we mentioned above.

Despite the absence of the serum from the Pasteur Institute in Lyon, Rabot was able to treat his first patient with the drug on October 15, 1894. A month after the announcement made by Emile Roux in Budapest, Rabot injected the two-year-old Jacques Cohen on the diphtheria ward (the *Salle Sainte Jeanne*) at the *Charité* using Behring's serum manufactured by Meister, Lucius and Brüning in Hoechst.[30] Rabot had been able to obtain limited quantities of German serum through Switzerland, but he complained that he could not apply the treatment regime he would have liked before the end of the year due to the scarcity and high cost of the drug. In the end, Rabot was able to start using the serum from the Pasteur Institute at the end of December 1894, and the Lyon serum produced by Arloing starting at the beginning of February 1895.[31]

The local history of Lyon has a number of features in common with other provincial towns. First, there is the significance of the Pasteur Institute's failure to supply the whole country after the nationwide publicity about the serum in September 1894. After January 1895, there were no new municipal initiatives to introduce local production as by this time there seems to have been a glut of serum rather than a lack. Second, serum production was regularly mobilized to further a wider bacteriological agenda in the region. While the city authorities demanded a reliable supply of serum to treat the local population, those charged with the mission often had grander ambitions. Gabriel Roux's project to expand Lyon's capacity for bacteriological analysis was typical of the kind of initiative built on the back of the demand for serum. In Lyon we also see the implication of the medical faculty because, although there was no teaching of bacteriology or microbiology at the time, those with the necessary skills were often associated with the medical school. As a result, as we shall see in the case of Nancy, teaching of bacteriology was often introduced into the city's medical school through the initiative to produce serum locally. Likewise, in Grenoble the introduction of local serum led in a relatively short time to the creation of a chair of microbiology at the medical faculty.

While the situation in Grenoble was in many respects similar to that in Lyon, the institutional response was somewhat different. The town was considerably smaller and it was close to Switzerland where it was possible to obtain the German serum. The archives in Grenoble provide more evidence of how the rarity of the serum penalized the provinces, with the Ministry of the Interior abetting the Pasteur Institute in its management of the penury. A telegram, from January 1895 to the Prefect of the *Isère* insists on the limited amount of serum that would be dispatched to the regional depots with the implicit privileging of Paris in the competition for supplies. Furthermore, it was the Prefect rather than the medical profession that would be charged with organizing the distribution of this new wonder drug.

> The depots of anti-diphtheria serum should be limited in number. The important thing is that you can obtain serum in case of need in some particular place in your department following the appearance of diphtheria. In order to do this, you should directly telegraph the Pasteur Institute, 21 rue Dutot.[32]

Such a telegram was doubtless intended simply to regulate the distribution of the serum by a form of rationing, but this kind of high-handed approach incited even smaller towns like Grenoble to undertake the production of their own serum.[33] Producing serum would allow the city to escape from its dependence on the Pasteur Institute, and, more importantly, the local supply of serum would no longer be managed by a centralized (Parisian) authority. In October 1894, Grenoble sent its Director of public health, Fernand Berlioz, to Paris to receive instruction on the preparation and use of serum at the Pasteur Institute. At the end of 1894, local fund-raising initiatives allowed the city to finance the purchase of five horses. Berlioz teamed up with Félix Jourdan director of the *Institut vaccinogène* to found the *Institut Sérothérapique* and, as in Lyon, they started producing anti-diphtheria serum in Grenoble in February 1895. The production was financed by the local authorities around the city, notably with the introduction of a 5 cent per head fee charged to these communities in order to have their own stock of serum.

Nevertheless, the Institute was nominally an independent private venture run by Berlioz and Jourdain who integrated the serum manufacture into their bacteriological analysis laboratory. The Dean of the Faculty of Medicine and Pharmacy in Grenoble was not happy with this situation and wanted the faculty to be more closely involved in the serum production. For him, it was unacceptable for the serum to be produced and sold by a private potentially for-profit Institute without appropriate supervision. In the end, the *Institut sérothérapique* was placed under the control of the city and the medical faculty, which was then allowed to use its facilities to teach bacteriology.[34]

The collaboration between the city and faculty via the *Institut sérothérapique* went even further, however, when in 1896 the city financed a chair of bacteriology and serotherapy at the faculty of medicine and pharmacy.[35] Once again, we can see a concrete example of how serum was a key factor in the introduction of the formal teaching of bacteriology in a medical school. While the form and financing of the serum producers in Lyon and Grenoble differed in their details, the overall principles were the same. The money for the facilities came from local subscriptions or municipal subsidies (not from private enterprise), and they were linked more or less closely to the medical faculty. In Lyon, the configuration of local public health politics and prominence of Gabriel Roux meant that the emphasis was placed on the development of a capacity for bacteriological diagnosis, whereas in Grenoble the faculty was more present, but the overall pattern confirms our argument about the wider influence of serum across France. Serum production was essentially viewed as a charitable rather than as a commercial venture, and local producers were obliged to conform to this image, often modeling their functioning on the Pasteur Institute in Paris. Paradoxically, however, their very existence countered the model of the Pasteur Institute, which from the beginning had positioned itself as the unique producer of anti-diphtheria serum in France. In Nancy, the city even went as far as to take money out of the Pasteur Institute's subscription to finance its own project.

Serum production in Nancy is a particularly significant case of this kind of local initiative, both because of the scale of the investment and because of the geopolitical situation of Nancy following the annexation of Alsace and Lorraine into the German Empire. After the capitulation of 1871, Nancy lay at the border with Germany, making it an important Nationalist symbol, physically marking the extent of France's perceived wound. These two aspects (financing and geopolitics) were related, as we shall see, but beyond these distinctive features, we can observe the same themes of local pride and medical education that we already saw in Lyon and Grenoble at work in Nancy.

Following the announcement in Budapest of Roux's success in treating diphtheria with the serum, the citizens of Nancy mobilized around the idea of having their own center to produce serum. To this end, local payments to the subscription for the Pasteur Institute were diverted to finance Nancy's own producer, the *Institut Sérothérapique de l'Est*.[36] On November 13, 1894, the organization committee composed of local dignitaries met in rooms belonging to the Society of Agriculture to discuss the plans for setting up the Institute. Three weeks later, on December 4, they met again at the town hall this time to discuss more detailed propositions. Meanwhile, a plan for a lottery had already been approved, with 1000 tickets to be sold at 25 centimes each. At the December meeting the committee drew up the statutes of the society that would run the institute. Five weeks later, on January 9, 1895, the *Institut sérothérapique de l'Est* was incorporated as a private, non-profit subscription company. The 11 initial shareholders—all prominent members of Nancy society, most with connections to the university—each pledged a non-refundable subscription of 100 francs to the Institute, providing a solid financial basis for its administration. The first president of the Institute was M. Alexandre-Alexis-Georges Le Monnier, a professor at the science faculty in Nancy, and deputy mayor.

From the outset the *Institut sérothérapique de l'Est* was independent but with strong attachments to the municipality, lying somewhere between the municipal structure set up in Lyon and the independent institution in Grenoble. The board governing the institute called in Eugène Macé, who occupied the chair of hygiene at the School of Medicine, to take care of the practical side of serum production. Macé had already been to Paris to work with Roux at the Pasteur Institute where he had learned the technique for producing serum, and he started the immunization process on a pair of horses at the end of 1894. The creation of the *Institut sérothérapique de l'Est* was followed in short order by a very generous anonymous donation of 40 000 francs. The money had been given specifically for the construction of a building to house the institute in Nancy. The anonymity of this gift was not maintained for very long and the donor was revealed to be the rich Parisian banker Daniel Iffla, also known as Osiris. The building, with the name Osiris prominently displayed above the main entrance opened its doors at the end of 1895. Unsurprisingly, considering the money involved, the completed building for the *Institut sérothérapique* was a lot more ambitious than its counterparts in Lyon or Grenoble. Although it only housed a pair of horses, it united diagnosis and production on a single site, and had space for a large lecture theater on the ground floor. With three laboratories on the first floor, the institute would combine teaching, research and production, positioning itself as a provincial exemplar of the model of the Pasteur Institut in Paris.

As with Lyon and Grenoble, Nancy started producing its own serum early in 1895, but once again this coincided with the period when the serum from the Pasteur Institute became readily available throughout France. This coincidence points to a profound irony of all these local ventures in serum production. Although the *Institut sérothérapique de l'Est* ended up distributing serum to Nancy and the surrounding area, in purely practical or economic terms, it turned out not to be necessary, and the same can be said for the facilities in Lyon, Grenoble and elsewhere. Limiting ourselves to the example of what happened in Nancy, should we dismiss this local institute and in particular the substantial investment in the Osiris building as a white elephant, or more generously put it down to a public health miscalculation? Either would, I believe, be an error, as serum from Paris was not the same as serum for Nancy for people living in the East of France. One central argument of this book has been that an important part of what constitutes a medical drug is what it means to people, patients (in this case, most often their families) and doctors alike. Thus, French serum was significantly different from British, Italian or German serum. In the same logic, serum from Nancy can be considered different from the serum produced by the Pasteur Institute in Paris. Although covered by the same national legislation, local production meant something to those who used the serum.

The building for the *Institut sérothérapique* was not the first gift that Osiris had made to the city of Nancy. A few years earlier he had paid for a statue of Joan of Arc. Facing east toward the annexed lands of the Lorraine, her standard raised high, she symbolized the French desire for revenge and the defense of the physical integrity of the Nation. Osiris's investment in the Institute and the production of serum in Nancy were of great symbolic value in France at the time. We have already seen how Rabot in Lyon switched from German to French serum as soon as possible, and this was not simply an economic choice as is suggested by his adoption of the Lyon serum once this became available.

In another sphere, that of the medical profession, we have seen how the local production of serum was bound into wider agendas of modernizing healthcare and medical training in cities like Lyon and Grenoble. Initially, serum gave access to financial resources that were then used for funding a range of bacteriological activities; it is evident that a new heroic medicine that saved children from the grip of diphtheria should raise more money than diagnostic tests or theoretical courses in the domain. We can see the appeal of serotherapy in the sheer range of fund-raising activities; special theater performances, tombolas and student-organized dances to name but three. It is clear, however, that in Nancy where only two horses were used to produce serum, the bulk of the money raised went into bacteriological testing with improved facilities and a larger capacity, microbiological research and teaching. By 1899, the *Institut sérothérapeutique de l'Est* was running out of steam, and became integrated into Nancy's Faculty of Medicine. The amphitheater was now officially for teaching bacteriology to medical students, whereas in the first 5 years of the institute's existence, its use for this purpose has been informal and voluntary.

It is important to understand the significance of using serum from Lyon, Grenoble, Bordeaux, Le Havre or Nancy as opposed to serum from Paris. Indeed, without a reflection on the political situation of France, it would be difficult to answer a simple question; why did the French even produce serum and not simply buy it from Germany? The aim here, however, is not to answer this question but to characterize a specifically French serum. Serum as a medical drug is an object that is constituted (at least in part) by its place of origin, although as with other medical drugs, particularly in the twentieth-century, the physical origin of the product is not generally considered important for evaluating its utility. While the battle between name-brand and generic drugs is fought over names and the connotations carried by these names (purity, reliability, quality), in the world of multinational pharmaceutical companies, the country of origin carries little weight.

To conclude this chapter on the regional producers of serum, we can note that there were some common characteristics shared by them all. Unlike the Pasteur Institute, they produced on a small scale to satisfy local demand, but like the Pasteur Istitute they were financed by a mix of charity and subsidies. The more or less intimate association of these producers with the medical schools set them apart from Paris, with the Pasteur Institute remaining staunchly independent. In general, the projects were entrusted to doctors who turned the interest in serum production toward the goal of building up bacteriology in the region. While this is interesting historical information in its own right, what does it tell us about serum as a technological object? Does it add anything that was not already presented in the analysis around Feenberg's schema of primary and secondary instrumentalization. I believe that it does, in at least two ways. First, the serum looks different as part of a struggle for local emancipation. Thus, serum produced in Lyon was not the same as the serum produced by the Pasteur Institute in Garches. This was not just a question of the label on the phial or the efficacy of the serum it contained (supposed or real). Injecting serum produced by Arloing in Lyon meant something different in the *Salle St Jeanne* at the *Charité* from using Roux's serum or a product from Germany, with local history and local feeling built into that difference.

Second, the serum and its production played an important role in local public health not just in the obvious sense of providing a treatment for a deadly disease, but by indirectly financing an infrastructure of bacteriological testing and education. This influx of money and interest offered the potential, at least in the domain of medical education, of putting regional centers ahead of Paris in this domain. While it would doubtless be an overstatement to say that using serotherapy (whether a national or local product) was conceived of as an act of patriotism by doctors and patients, there was something different and special about French serum as there was about serum from Lyon or from Nancy.

NOTES

1. Gaston Calmette, 'La Guérison du Croup à l'Institut Pasteur.' *Le Figaro* (September 6, 1894) p.1. C'est donc une oeuvre française, exclusivement française, puisque, partie tout d'abord de l'Institut de la rue Dutot, et essayée ensuite à l'étranger, c'est dans ce même Institut de la rue Dutot qu'elle vient prendre, auprès des mêmes hommes, son perfectionnement définitif et son dernier essor.

2. Anon. 'Voilà donc cette barbare diphtérie, le fléau des enfants, la terreur des mères à peu près vaincue grâce aux patientes recherches du Docteur Roux, l'infatigable élève du Grand Pasteur.' Archives de l'Institut Pasteur, folder Emile Roux.

3. Louis Pasteur was imbued early on with a strong sense of patriotism by his father who had spent his youth fighting in Napoleon's army. Today, however, this side of Pasteur's reputation is much less well known, with his reputation as the 'bienfaiteur de l'humanité' resting primarily on his treatment for rabies.

4. Louis Pasteur, *Quelques réflexions sur la science en France* (Paris, France: Gauthier-Villars, 1871), p. 26. Originally published in the *Salut Public* in March 1871. 'Je me propose de démontrer dans cet écrit que si, au moment du péril suprême, la France n'a pas trouvé des hommes supérieurs pour mettre en œuvre ses ressources et le courage de ses enfants, il faut l'attribuer, j'en ai la conviction, à ce que la France s'est désintéressée, depuis un demi-siècle, des grands travaux de la pensée, particulièrement dans les sciences exactes.'

5. I am talking of the popular success of the rabies vaccine rather than its 'success' in terms of the number of lives saved. For a detailed assessment of the clinical virtues and vices of the vaccine, see Gerald Geison, *The Private Science of Louis Pasteur*, (Princeton: Princeton University Press, 1995).

6. *Le Salut Public*, vendredi 16 novembre 1888.

7. For an overview of the development of these missions, see Ilana Lowy, 'On Hybridizations, Networks, and New Disciplines: The Pasteur Institute and the Development of Microbiology in France,' *Studies in the History and Philosophy of Science*, 1994, 655–88.

8. Harriette Chick, Margaret Hume and Marjorie Macfarlane, *War on Disease: a History of the Lister Institute* (London: Deutsch, 1971).

9. Ibid, pp. 30–1.

10. Roy Church and Elizabeth Tansey, *Burroughs, Wellcome & Co. : Knowledge, Trust, Profit and the Transformation of the British Pharmaceutical Industry, 1880–1940* (Lancaster: Crucible, 2007).

11. Paul Weindling, 'Scientific Elites and Laboratory Organisation in Fin de Siècle Paris and Berlin. The Pasteur Institute and Robert Koch Institute for Infectious Diseases Compared,' in Andrew Cunningham and Perry Williams (eds), *The Laboratory Revolution in Medicine* (Cambridge: Cambridge University Press, 1992), 170–88.

12. The prominence of Moizard in this public demonstration of the serotherapy could only have heightened Roux's sense of betrayal the following year. See chapter 6.

13. *Le Figaro*, October 24, 1894.

14. For more on this episode, see Christoph Gradmann, *Laboratory Disease: Robert Koch's Medical Bacteriology* (Baltimore: Johns Hopkins University Press, 2009)

15. In the French pharmaceutical legislation dating from 1803, there was not even an explicit definition of a medical drug. The law granted the monopoly of the sale of medical drugs to the pharmacists in return for their agreement to limit their commerce to these products. Nevertheless, medical drugs were taken to correspond to the list found in the official pharmacopeia plus preparations carried out in accordance with the explicit directions of a doctor's prescription. Serum, like vaccines answered to neither of these definitions. See 'Loi contenant organisation des écoles de pharmacie 21 germinal de l'an XI' *Bulletin des Lois*, 3e série, no 270, p. 121. (11 avril 1803)

16. I do not intend to use the adjective 'fringe' in a perjorative sense, I just want to underline that both vaccination and the various opotherapies of the time were at the margins of mainstream medicine. *Journal Officiel*, 12 avril 1895, documents parlementaires, chambre des députés, p. 313. Article 14 of the pharmacy law that was under debate in 1895 was the original legislative tool (The text is to be found in the *Annexe Journal Officiel, Documents Parlementaires, Chambre des députés*, 10 janvier 1895, p. 1–3, art 9 on p. 1 and art 14 pp. 1–2)

17. *Journal officiel du 30 janvier 1895*, annexe p. 2. The text also excluded the smallpox vaccine from the law.

18. Article 1 of the law of April 25, 1895. The addition of the last category took aim at the practice of opotherapy, the medical use of extracts of animal organs popularized by Brown-Séquard. For more on Brown-Séquard, see Merriley Borell 'Brown-Séquard's organotherapy and its appearance in America at the end of the nineteenth century,' *Bulletin of the History of Medicine*, 50.3 (1976), pp. 309–320.

19. 'Discussion d'un projet de loi relative aux serums thérapeutiques' Séance du 6 avril 1895, *Journal Officiel*, 1895 annexe, p. 1229.

20. *Journal Officiel*, 4 mars 1895, documents parlementaires, p. 247

21. It seems that only fifteen of the projected sixteen members were appointed: Brouardel, Monod, Proust, Chantemesse, Bompard, Delaunay-Belleville, Bergeron (Secretaries of the Académie de médecine), Nocard, Duclaux, Straus, Grancher (ordinary members of the Académie de médecine), and Pouchet, Ogier, Thoinot, Netter (Members of the Comité consultatif d'hygiène).

22. While the Pasteur Institute in Lille, run by Albert Calmette was nominally independent, it functioned as a subsidiary of the Paris institution.

23. In addition there were two approved producers of opotherapies (organic extracts prepared according to Brown-Séquard's method), one in Paris (Laboratoire de MM. Egasse et Bouyé, rue des Fossés-Saint-Jacques) and the other in Bordeaux (Laboratoire de M. Bazin, cours Victor-Hugo).

24. *Salut Public*, September 7, 1894, p. 1.

25. François Rabot, 'Prélude à la sérothérapie,' *Lyon médical*, 77 (1894), pp. 527–43, on p. 538.

26. Archives de l'Institut Pasteur, Direction (1888–1940) File 'Création du service de sérothérapie.'

27. Note, Registre de l'Hôpital des Enfants-Malades, 18 octobre 1894, Archives de l'Assistance Publique—Hôpitaux de Paris, pp. 292–3. 'J'ai informé M. Gallet que les enfants de la province affluaient à l'hôpital pour bénéficier du traitement de M. le Dr. Roux, et qu'il fallait prévoir, à courte écheance, un encombrement du service de

la diphtérie. M. Gallet m'a autorisé à ouvrir une salle de huit lits sous la crèche, et à faire payer les enfants qui seraient en situation de la faire.'

28. Report 'Rapport de M. le Dr. Roux soumis à Monsieur le Maire,' November 6, 1894, Archives Municipales de Lyon 1125 WP 023 2.

29. Report to the Mayor of Lyon by Gabriel Roux, January 29, 1895, Archives Municipales, Lyon.

30. François Rabot, 'Prélude à la sérothérapie,' p. 539.

31. Perre Patet, 'La sérothérapie à Lyon' (MD thesis, Lyon Faculty of Medicine, 1895).

32. Telegram from the Ministry of the Interior to the Prefects of France, January 28, 1895 (Archives départementales de l'Isère, folder 114 M1)

33. In 1896 Grenoble had a population of 64 000 compared to Lyon's population of 466 000 (or Nancy, 96 000)

34. More details are available in a PhD dissertation on public health policy in the Isère; Lucie Paquy, 'Santé publique et pouvoirs locaux. Le département de l'Isère et la loi du 15 février 1902.' (Université Lyon 2, 2001).

35. Archives Departementales de l'Isère file 2T8

36. See Pierre Parisot, 'L'Institut sérothérapique de l'Est contre la diphtérie' *Revue médicale de l'Est*, vol. 26 (1894), p. 692, where Parisot (a leading figure in medicine, particularly bacteriology in Nancy and editor of the journal) announces that the subscription conducted by this journal would go to the local *Institut de l'Est* rather than to the Pasteur Institute.

Chapter 9

Conclusion

After seven chapters on the history of one single pharmaceutical product in one country over a relatively short period of time (1894–1900), we can perhaps begin to formulate an answer to the more general question with which we started this book. What can we learn from approaching a medical drug like serum as a technological object? With our relatively narrow focus, we have been able to spread the French serum out across the pages of this book in a process akin to the anatomical dissection, with each chapter bringing a different aspect of this drug to the fore. While we started with the very material questions of the production and preparation of the antitoxin, by the third and fourth chapters our attention had turned to contextual elements that gave shape to the serum, like the legislation covering the drug or the mortality statistics used to demonstrate its efficacy. The successive chapters illustrated how the serotherapy was integrated at different levels of medical and administrative systems, with the law of 1895 covering sera and vaccines a particularly striking example of how the serum in turn transformed these very systems. The motivation behind presenting all these elements from the material to the legal, social and political is to advance the claim that they are all constitutive of the serum. If there is one lesson that we can draw from the philosophy of technology since the 1960s it is that a technological object is not simply a material object in use or the technological solution to a practical problem, but that the object is given form and sense through the context in which it is adopted and the multiple roles it fulfills.

As it was informed by political and professional interests, the serum also acted in return. We have suggested, although not analyzed in detail the ways in which this innovative drug contributed to shaping French medicine and ’en society at the end of the nineteenth century.

The entry into this subject via the philosophy of technology allows us to read the history differently from the classic model in the history of pharmacy. Our approach has drawn attention to the integration of a complex set of elements that would not have been visible had we limited our investigation to the development of the first sera and the history of their clinical use, or even if we had opened the investigation up to questions of industrial production. Indeed, although I consider myself a historian of science, I am tempted to make the disloyal observation that the greatest advantage of treating serum as a technological object rather than as a historical subject has been the unhistorical nature of the resulting analysis. Here, I do not mean that the study has been a-historical in the derogatory sense in which historians use this term. When historians talk of an a-historical approach, they are pointing to the universalizing, timeless nature of the analysis, a pretention to a 'view from nowhere' in a case where a specific historical episode is taken to illustrate a universal truth. While there is, of course, some risk of this in presenting a medical drug as a technological object, here I just wanted to underline how the presentation of serum in this book does not conform to the norms of historical narrative. In general, histories of drugs, irrespective of whether they focus on the 'science,' the 'social' or find themselves somewhere in between, are oriented toward the trajectories of these drugs across time, close to the model of biographies for living historical figures. The classic format involves recounting the discovery, development, and, in some cases, the marketing, consumption or even demise of the drug under consideration.[1] While we did present some of the elements of the beginnings of serotherapy, we did not go into detail concerning this research,[2] and the fate of the serotherapy in the twentieth century was left completely to one side.

Rather than presenting this kind of history, the study in this book has offered something closer to a synchronic slice, looking at how the serum was deployed across different spaces—from the laboratory of the Pasteur Institute to the hospital setting (as in the *Charité* hospital in Lyon), as well as considering serum production in the provinces. This work is historical, because the serum was introduced over a century ago and passed out of current use some fifty years later, but it does not conform to a classic historical narrative. The fact that the book is not structured by a beginning and a rise (and, as often as not, a fall) brings other elements into focus, notably the association with other technologies and contemporary social, professional and political structures. One such aspect is the importance of the relationship between serotherapy and microbiology in France. In contrast to certain histories of medicine that vaunt the triumph of Louis Pasteur in introducing the germ theory to French medicine, we have seen that serotherapy—introduced while Pasteur was on his deathbed—was instrumental in engaging large numbers of doctors in an active study (and practice) of microbiology and provided the concrete means for introducing this subject into medical schools across France. [3] But our analysis of serotherapy has taken us well beyond the issue of the place of microbiology in France. We have seen how serum tapped into deep structures within French society, such as the place of women in the workforce and the social perspective on women's relationship to children and care as well as the changing perception of the medical profession. The full sense of serotherapy also depended on more contingent fluctuating historical features of late nineteenth-century France, such as the after-effects of the Franco-Prussian war and the repercussions of a period of rapid industrialization.

The most glaring gap in our presentation of serotherapy and diphtheria is on the side of the experience of the patient and the relationship between patient, doctor and family around the serum. This is due to a lack of sources, as we found it practically impossible to uncover consistent evidence concerning these relationships from the publications and archives we consulted. This suggests that the present work could be usefully complemented by a study of the use of a contemporary medical drug, as it is difficult to get an idea of how people see and understand medicines without interviewing them or devising some other means for obtaining this information directly from the patient.[4] It is perhaps symptomatic of our modern attitude to medical drugs that this kind of data has not been collected and does not appear to be a priority for the producers, prescribers and financers of such drugs, even today. Anthropology is much more concerned with the use of illegal recreational drugs than the millions of medical drugs prescribed every day. Despite this missing element, the synchronic picture of the serum at the end of the nineteenth century is not without interest for those oriented toward the social history of medicine, and, unlike many histories of drugs, is not exclusively focused on the scientists who invented and manufactured it.

But what does this study of an atypical technological object tell us about technology, or more precisely what can the philosophy of technology gain from this work? Right at the beginning I pointed out that medical drugs, and serum in particular, are not the first things that come to mind when we are asked to think of a technological object. Nevertheless, there is no good reason to discount the serum, or any other medical drug, as a technology. Indeed, recent work on human enhancement aligns drugs (mainly through the phenomenon of doping) with other more intuitively obvious candidates for technological objects, like prostheses, within a spectrum of enhancement technologies. Once again, a medical drug is quite different from a machine, a computing device, or even a carbon-fiber prosthetic limb. The real advantage of considering a medical drug in terms of technology is that this approach gives it a status that allows us to think about the object instead of looking on it as a transparent delivery system for a physiological effect. Rather than thinking of serum as something for curing diphtheria (as one might think of aspirin as something for treating a headache) we have tried our best to displace it from this logic and have been looking at its meaning as a product, placing the supposed physiological property on a similar analytical plane with its mode of distribution or financing. Of course, while I have been arguing that all these elements contribute to the meaning of the drug, I do not want to suggest that they all contribute in the same way or to the same degree.

As I have just explained, this book does not read like a classic historical presentation of a drug, and the philosophical question that underwrites my approach might make it seem unsatisfying to historians. Nevertheless, this book does not read like a classic philosophical treatise either. Once again, I hope that this does not put philosophers of science and technology off, as there are profound philosophical lessons that the reader can take away from this analysis. First, that to understand what technology is and how it works we need to consider a wider range of examples than those standardly taken into account. Second, that to understand a technological object we need to look at a broad range of domains and not limit ourselves to an analysis of its mechanical function in the world. Last, but not least, the reflexive lesson that serotherapy teaches us once again is that our modern societies (and probably pre-modern societies as well) are as much a product of the technologies that they deploy as they are the authors and masters of these technologies. This is as true for medical drugs as it is for mobile phones or laptop computers. If the next time you take a pill or receive a vaccine you think of serum and its multilayered meanings, this analysis will have served a purpose.

NOTES

1. As examples of the various approaches, we can cite an excellent history of amphetamines, Nicolas Rasmussen, *On Speed: The Many Lives of Amphetamine* (New York: NYU Press, 2009), and the very narrative-driven history of Penicillin by Robert Bud, *Penicillin: Triumph and* Tragedy (Oxford University Press, 2007).

2. I have presented this subject in an article, Jonathan Simon, 'Emil Behring's medical culture: from disinfection to serotherapy.' *Medical History* 51 (2007): 201–18.

3. Michael Worboys's detailed investigation of the uptake of germ theory suggests that doctors' interest in Britain was likewise indexed on the utility of the theory rather than constituting a revelation inspired by pure science. Michael Worboys, *Spreading Germs: Disease Theories and Medical Practice in Britain, 1865–1900* (Cambridge: Cambridge University Press, 2000).

4. See Sylvie Fainzang, *Médicaments et sociétés, le patient, le médecin et l'ordonnance* (Paris: Presses Universitaires de France, 2001).

Bibliography

Akrich, Madeleine. 'Petite anthropologie du médicament.' *Techniques et Culture*, 1995, 129–57.

Aristotle. *The Physics*. Translated by Philip Henry Wicksteed and Francis Macdonald Cornford. 2 vols. Cambridge: Harvard University Press, 1957.

Aschkinazi, Eugène. 'Le Stérésol (vernis antiseptique) et ses applications spécialement dans la diphtérie.' Faculté de Médecine de Paris, 1893.

Behring, Emil, and Shibasaburo Kitasato. 'Ueber das Zustandekommen der Diphtherie-Immunität und der Tetanus-Immunität bei Thieren.' *Deutsche Medicinische Wochenscrift*, no. 49 (1890): 1113–14.

Bijker, Wiebe E. *Of Bicycles, Bakelites, and Bulbs: Toward a Theory of Sociotechnical Change*. Cambridge MA: The MIT Press, 1997.

Bloor, David. *Knowledge and Social Imagery*. London: Routledge & Kegan Paul, 1976.

Borell, Merriley. 'Brown-Séquard's Organotherapy and its Appearance in America at the End of the Nineteenth Century.' *Bulletin of the History of Medicine* 50, no. 3 (1976): 309–20.

Bud, Robert. *Penicillin: Triumph and Tragedy*. Oxford University Press, 2007.

Calmette, Gaston. 'La Guérison du croup à l'Institut Pasteur.' *Le Figaro*, September 6, 1894.

Carnap, Rudolf. *Der Logische Aufbau der Welt*. Berlin, Allemagne: Schlachtensee Welkreis-Verlag, 1928.

Chary, Victor. 'La Mortalité par diphtérie en Europe avant et après l'application de la sérothérapie (étude statistique).' Faculté de Médecine de Paris, 1900.

Chast, François. *Histoire contemporaine des médicaments*. Paris: La Découverte, 2002.

Chauveau, *L'Invention pharmaceutique: la pharmacie française entre l'état et la société au XXe siècle*. Les Empêcheurs de penser en rond. Paris: Sanofi-Synthélabo, 1999.

Chick, Harriette, Eleanor Hume, and Marjorie Macfarlane. *War on Disease: A History of the Lister Institute*. London: Deutsch, 1971.

Church, Roy, and Elizabeth Tansey. *Burroughs, Wellcome & Co.: Knowledge, Trust, Profit and the Transformation of the British Pharmaceutical Industry, 1880–1940.* Lancaster: Crucible, 2007.

Close-Koenig, Tricia. 'Betwixt and Between. Production and Commodification of Knowledge in a Medical School Pathological Anatomy Laboratory, Strasbourg (Mid-19th Century to 1939).' University of Strasbourg, 2011.

Cobbett, Louis. 'Has Antitoxine reduced the Death Rate from Diphtheria in Our Large Towns?' *Edinburgh Medical Journal*, 1900.

Colgrove, James. 'The McKeown Thesis: A Historical Controversy and Its Enduring Influence.' *American Journal of Public Health* 92, no. 5 (May 2002): 725–29.

Cowan, Ruth Schwartz. *A Social History of American Technology.* New York ; Oxford: Oxford University Press, 1997.

Dracobly, Alex. 'Ethics and Experimentation on Human Subjects in Mid-Nineteenth-Century France: The Story of the 1859 Syphilis Experiments.' *Bulletin of the History of Medicine* 77, no. 2 (2003): 332–66.

Ducassé, Pierre. *Les techniques et le philosophe.* Paris: Presses Universitaires de France, 1958.

Dusek, Val. *Philosophy of Technology: An Introduction.* Oxford: Blackwell, 2006.

Earles, Melvin. 'Early Theories of the Mode of Action of Drugs and Poisons.' *Annals of Science* 17, no. 2 (1961): 97–110.

Egarter, Christian, Christoph Grimm, Kazem Nouri, Hans-Joachim Ahrendt, Johannes Bitzer, and Christine Cermak. 'Contraceptive Counselling and Factors Affecting Women's Contraceptive Choices: Results of the CHOICE Study in Austria.' *Reproductive Biomedicine Online* 24, no. 7 (June 2012): 692–97. doi:10.1016/j.rbmo.2011.12.003.

Ehrlich, Paul. 'Die Wertbemessung des Diphtherieheilserums und deren theoretische Grundlagen.' *Klinisches Jahrbuch* 6 (1897): 299–326.

Ehrlich, Paul Ralph. *The collected papers of Paul Ehrlich.* Edited by F. Himmelweit, Martha Marquardt, and Henry Hallett Dale. London: Pergamon, 1956.

Fainzang, Sylvie. *Médicaments et sociétés, le patient, le médecin et l'ordonnance.* Paris: Presses Universitaires de France, 2001.

Fayssoil, Abdallah. 'René Laennec (1781–1826) and the Invention of the Stethoscope.' *The American Journal of Cardiology* 104, no. 5 (September 1, 2009): 743–44. doi:10.1016/j.amjcard.2009.06.053.

Feenberg, Andrew. *Questioning Technology*. London: Routledge, 1999.

Fishman, Jennifer R. 'Making Viagra: From Impotence to Erectile Dysfunction.' In *Medicating Modern America*, edited by Andrea Tone and Elizabeth Siegel Watkins, 229–52. New York: New York University Press, 2007.

Funck, M. *Manuel de sérothérapie antidiphtérique*. Paris: Carré, 1895.

Gachelin, Gabriel. 'The Building up of a Culture of Standardization at the Institut Pasteur, 1885–1900.' *HAL, Web Open Archives* halshs-00335350 (n.d.): 2008.

Gardey, Delphine. *La dactylographe et l'expéditionnaire: histoire des employés de bureau: 1890–1930*. Paris: Belin, 2001.

Gardner, Paula. 'Distorted Packaging: Marketing Depression as Illness, Drugs as Cure.' *Journal of Medical Humanities* 24, no. 1–2 (June 1, 2003): 105–30. doi:10.1023/A:1021314017235.

Geison, Gerald L. *The Private Science of Louis Pasteur*. Princeton: Princeton University Press, 1995.

Goethe, Johann Wolfgang von. *Faust*. DigBib.Org: Die digitale Bibliothek., 2004.

Goldstein, Jan. *Console and Classify: The French Psychiatric Profession in the Nineteenth Century*. Chicago: University of Chicago Press, 2001.

Goodman, Jordan, Paul E. Lovejoy, and Andrew Sherratt, eds. *Consuming Habits: Drugs in History and Anthropology*. London: Routledge, 1995.

Goubeau, and J. Hulot. 'Traitement de l'angine diphtéritique par les badigeonnages du fond de la gorge avec une solution concentrée de sublimé dans la glycérine.' *Archives Générales de Médecine* 8, no. 2 (1894): 289–418.

Gradmann, Christoph. *Laboratory Disease: Robert Koch's Medical Bacteriology*. Baltimore: Johns Hopkins University Press, 2009.

Gradmann, Christoph, and Jonathan Simon, eds. *Evaluating and Standardizing Therapeutic Agents, 1890–1950*. Basingstoke: Palgrave Macmillan, 2010.

Greene, Jeremy A. *Prescribing by Numbers: Drugs and the Definition of Disease*. Baltimore: The Johns Hopkins University Press, 2006.

Greene, Jeremy A, and Elizabeth Siegel Watkins. *Prescribed: Writing, Filling, Using, and Abusing the Prescription in Modern America*. Baltimore: The Johns Hopkins University Press, 2012.

Hardy, Anne. *The Epidemic Streets: Infectious Diseases and the Rise of Preventive Medicine 1856–1900*. Oxford: Clarendon Press, 1993.

Hardy, Anne I. 'From Diphtheria to Tetanus: The Development of Evaluation Methods for Sera in Imperial Germany.' In *Evaluating and Standardizing Therapeutic Agents, 1890–1950*, edited by Christoph Gradmann and Jonathan Simon. Basingstoke: Palgrave Macmillan, 2010, 52–70.

Hess, David J. *Science Studies: An Advanced Introduction*. New York: New York University Press, 1997.

Hess, Volker. *Der wohltemperierte Mensch: Wissenschaft und Alltag des Fiebermessens (1850–1900)*. Frankfurt am Main: Campus Verlag, 2000.

Home, Francis. *An Inquiry into the Nature, Cause, and Cure of the Croup*. Edinburgh: A. Kincaid and J. Bell, 1765.

Howell, Joel D. *Technology in the Hospital: Transforming Patient Care in the Early Twentieth Century*. Baltimore: The Johns Hopkins University Press, 1996.

Hüntelmann, Axel. 'Diphtheria Serum and Serotherapy. Development, Production and Regulation in Fin de Siècle Germany.' *Dynamis* 27 (2007): 107–31.

———. 'The Anti-Diphtheria Serum and the Case of Langerhans.' *Medizin, Gesellschaft, und Geschichte: Jahrbuch des Instituts für Geschichte der Medizin der Robert Bosch Stiftung* 24 (2005): 71–104.

Illich, Ivan. *Energy and Equity*. New York: Marion Boyars, 1974.

———. *Medical Nemesis: The Expropriation of Health*. New York: Pantheon Books, 1976.

Kapp, Ernst. *Grundlinien einer Philosophie der Technik: zur Entstehungsgeschichte der Cultur aus neuen Gesichtspunkten*. Braunschweig: G. Westermann, 1877.

Katz, James Everett, ed. *Machines That Become Us: The Social Context of Personal Communication Technology*. New Brunswick NJ: Transaction Publishers, 2003.

Kocturk, Tahire O. 'Food Rules in the Koran.' *Food & Nutrition Research* 46, no. 3 (September 1, 2002): 137–39. doi:10.3402/fnr.v46i3.1451.

Kruif, Paul de. *Microbe Hunters*. New York: Kessinger Publishing, 1926.

Landouzy, Louis. *Les sérothérapies: leçons de thérapeutique et matière médicale, professées à la Faculté de Médecine de l'Université de Paris*. Paris: G. Carré et C. Naud, 1898.

Latour, Bruno. 'Give Me a Laboratory and I Will Move the World.' In *Science Observed*, edited by Karin Knorr-Cetina and Michael Mulkay, London: Sage, 1983, 141–70.

———. *The Pasteurization of France*. Harvard University Press, 1993.

Lecourt, Dominique. *La philosophie des sciences*. Paris: Presses universitaires de France, 2010.

Lemière, Georges. *La diphtérie et son traitement par la sérumthérapie*. Lille: L. Danel, 1895.

Lemieux, Raymond, and Ulrike Spohr. 'How Emil Fischer Was Led to the Lock and Key Concept for Enzyme Specificity.' In *Advances in Carbohydrate Chemistry and Biochemistry*, San Diego: Academic Press, 1994, 1–19.

Loeffler, Friedrich. 'Untersuchung über die Bedeutung der Mikroorganismen für die Entstehung der Diphtherie.' *Mitteilungen des kaiserlichen Gesundheitsamtes* 2 (1884): 421–99.

Lowy, Ilana. 'On Hybridizations, Networks, and New Disciplines: The Pasteur Institute and the Development of Microbiology in France.' *Studies in the History and Philosophy of Science*, 1994.

Madsen, Thorvald. 'Ueber Messung der Stärke des antidiphtherischen Serums.' *Zeitschrift für Hygiene und Infektionskrankheiten* 24 (1897): 425–42.

Maehle, Andreas-Holger. *Drugs on Trial: Experimental Pharmacology and Therapeutic Innovation in the Eighteenth Century*. The Wellcome Institute series in the history of medicine. Amsterdam: Rodopi, 1999.

Martin, Louis. 'Production de la toxine diphtérique.' Faculté de Médecine de Paris, 1897.

Mazumdar, Pauline M. H. 'The State, the Serum Institutes and the League of Nations.' in *Evaluating and Standardizing Therapeutic Agents, 1890–1950*, edited by Christoph Gradmann and Jonathan Simon, 118–38. Basingstoke: Palgrave Macmillan, 2010.

McKeown, Thomas. *Medicine in Modern Society*. London: George Allen and Unwin, 1965.

Mendelsohn, Andrew. 'Cultures of Bacteriology: Formation and Transformation of a Science in France and Germany, 1870–1914.' Princeton University, 1996.

———. 'The Microscopist of Modern Life.' *Osiris* 18 (January 1, 2003): 150–70.

Mercier, R. 'A Propos des indications et des accidents de la sérothérapie antidiphtérique.' *La Semaine médicale*, 1896.

Merton, Robert. 'The Normative Structure of Science.' In *The Sociology of Science: Theoretical and Empirical Investigations*, Chicago: University of Chicago Press, 1979, 1–19.

Mitcham, Carl. *Thinking through Technology: The Path between Engineering and Philosophy*. Chicago: University of Chicago Press, 1994.

Moizard, Paul, and Bouchard. 'Un cas d'angine non-diphtérique traité par le sérum suivi de mort,' *Bulletins et mémoires de la Société médicale des hôpitaux de Paris*, 1895, 525–34.

Paquy, Lucie. 'Santé publique et pouvoirs locaux. Le département de l'Isère et la loi du 15 février 1902.' Université Lyon 2, 2001.

Parisot, Pierre. 'L'Institut sérothérapique de l'Est contre la diphtérie' *Revue médicale de l'Est*, vol. 26 (1894): 692–93.

Pasteur, Louis. *Quelques réflexions sur la science en France*. Paris, France: Gauthier-Villars, 1871.

Patet, Pierre. 'La Sérothérapie à Lyon.' Faculté de Médecine de Lyon, 1895.

Persy, Paul. *Ma première application du sérum antidiphtérique*. Le Mans: Monnoyer, 1895.

Phily, F. *Jurisprudence générale et législation de la Médecine-pharmacie, à l'usage des médecins, chirurgiens, pharmaciens, dentistes, sages-femmes, vétérinaires, herboristes. Décisions de toutes les juridictions . . . publiées depuis quinze ans (1895–1910) . . . suivies de la législation, réunies, classées et présentées par MM. F. Phily* aîné, . . . Henri *Petel . . . F. Izouard, . . . avec le concours de MM. A. Crinon, Marcel Petit et P. Bogelot,* . . . Paris: Administration du Recueil des sommaires de la jurisprudence francaise, 1911.

Pinch, Trevor, and Wiebe Bijker. 'The Social Construction of Facts and Artefacts: Or How the Sociology of Science and the Sociology of Technology Might Benefit Each Other.' *Social Studies of Science* 14 (1984): 399–441.

Pitt, Joseph C. *Doing Philosophy of Technology: Essays in a Pragmatist Spirit*. Dordrecht: Springer, 2011.

Porter, Roy. 'The Patient's View: Doing Medical History from Below.' *Theory and Society* 14, no. 2 (1985): 175–98.

Prüll, Cay-Rudiger. 'Paul Ehrlich's Standardization of Serum: Wertbestimmung and Its Meaning for Twentieth-Century Biomedicine.' In *Evaluating and Standardizing Therapeutic Agents, 1890–1950*, edited by Christoph Gradmann and Jonathan Simon, Basingstoke: Palgrave Macmillan, 2010, 13–30.

Rabot, François. 'Prélude à la sérothérapie.' *Lyon médical* 77 (1894): 527–543.

Rasmussen, Anne. 'Les enjeux d'une histoire des formes pharmaceutiques: La galénique, l'officine et l'industrie (XIXe—début XXe siècle).' *Entreprises et histoire* n° 36, no. 2 (June 1, 2004): 12–28.

Rasmussen, Nicolas. *On Speed: The Many Lives of Amphetamine*. New York: NYU Press, 2009.

Robinson, Daniel H, and Alexander H Toledo. 'Historical Development of Modern Anesthesia.' *Journal of Investigative Surgery: The Official Journal of the Academy of Surgical Research* 25, no. 3 (June 2012): 141–49. doi:10.3109/08941939.2012.690328.

Roche, Daniel. *La culture équestre occidentale, XVIe-XIXe siècle: l'ombre du cheval*. Paris: Fayard, 2008.

Roux, Émile. 'A Propos d'une observation de MM. Moizard et Bouchard sur un cas d'angine non-diphtérique traité par le sérum et suivi de mort,' *Journal de clinique et de thérapeutique infantiles* 3, no. 31 (1895): 601.

———. 'Discours de M. le Dr Roux, Directeur de l'Institut Pasteur.' in *Edmond Nocard 1850–1903, discours prononcés à la cérémonie d'inauguration du monument élevé à sa mémoire*. Paris: Masson et cie, n.d.

Roux, Émile, and Louis Martin. 'Contribution à l'étude de la diphtérie (sérum-thérapie).' *Annales de l'Institut Pasteur* 8, no. 9 (1894): 609–39.

Roux, Émile, and Alexandre Yersin. 'Contribution à l'étude de la diphthérie.' *Annales de l'Institut Pasteur* 2, no. 12 (1888): 629–61.

Ruud, Johan T. 'Vertebrates without Erythrocytes and Blood Pigment.' *Nature* 173, no. 4410 (May 8, 1954): 848–50. doi:10.1038/173848a0.

Schlich, Thomas. *The Origins of Organ Transplantation: Surgery and Laboratory Science, 1880–1930*. Rochester: University of Rochester Press, 2010.

Schulte, Erika. 'Der Anteil Erich Wernickes an der Entwicklung des Diphtherieantitoxins.' der Freie Universität Berlin, 2000.

Silverstein, Arthur. *A History of Immunology*. San Diego: Academic Press, 1989.

Simon, Jonathan. *Chemistry, Pharmacy and Revolution*. Aldershot: Ashgate, 2005.

———. 'Emil Behring's Medical Culture: From Disinfection to Serotherapy.' *Medical History* 51 (April 2007): 201–18.

———. 'Monitoring the Stable at the Pasteur Institute.' *Science in Context* 21, no. 2 (2008): 181–200. doi:10.1017/S0269889708001683.

———. 'Standardization and Clinical Use: The Introduction of the Anti-Diphtheria Serum in Lyon.' In *Biologics: A History of Agents Made from Living Organisms in the Twentieth Century*, edited by Alexander von Schwerin, Heiko Stoff, and Bettina Wahrig, 33–46. London: Pickering & Chatto, 2013.

Simon, Jules (1831–1899). *Nouvelles études sur la diphtérie, par le Dr Jules Simon, . . .* Paris: Masson, 1889.

Sinding, Christiane. 'Making the Unit of Insulin: Standards, Clinical Work and Industry, 1920–1925.' *Bulletin of the History of Medicine* 76, no. 2 (2002): 231–70.

Tauber, Alfred I., and Leon Chernyak. *Metchnikoff and the Origins of Immunology: From Metaphor to Theory*. Monographs on the history and philosophy of biology, Oxford: Oxford University Press, 1991.

Thoinot, Léon-Henri, and E.-Jules Masselin. *Précis de microbie médicale et vétérinaire*. Paris: G. Masson, 1889.

Throm, Carola. *Das Diphtherieserum: ein neues Therapieprinzip, seine Entwicklung und Markteinfuhrung*. Heidelberg: Wissenschaftliche Verlagsgesellschaft, 1995.

Timmermann, Carsten, and Julie Anderson, eds. *Devices and Designs: Medical Technologies in Historical Perspective*. Houndmills: Palgrave Macmillan, 2006.

Timmermans, Stefan, and Marc Berg. *The Gold Standard: The Challenge of Evidence-Based Medicine and Standardization in Health Care*. Philadelphia: Temple University Press, 2003.

Turkle, Sherry. *Alone Together: Why We Expect More from Technology and Less from Each Other*. New York: Basic Books, 2011.

———. *The Second Self: Computers and the Human Spirit*. Cambridge MA: MIT Press, 2005.

Turkle, Sherry, and Seymour Papert. 'Epistemological Pluralism: Styles and Voices within the Computer Culture.' *Signs* 16, no. 1 (October 1, 1990): 128–57. doi:10.2307/3174610.

Vares, Tiina, and Virginia Braun. 'Spreading the Word, but What Word Is That? Viagra and Male Sexuality in Popular Culture.' *Sexualities* 9, no. 3 (January 7, 2006): 315–32. doi:10.1177/1363460706065055.

Watkins, Elizabeth Siegel. *On the Pill: A Social History of Oral Contraceptives, 1950–1970.* Baltimore: Johns Hopkins University Press, 2001.

Weindling, Paul. 'From Medical Research to Clinical Practice: Serum Therapy for Diphtheria in the 1890s.' In *Medical Innovations in Historical Perspective*, edited by John Pickstone, New York: St Martin's Press, 1992, 72–83.

———. 'Scientific Elites and Laboratory Organisation in Fin de Siècle Paris and Berlin. The Pasteur Institute and Robert Koch Institute for Infectious Diseases Compared.' In *The Laboratory Revolution in Medicine*, edited by Andrew Cunningham and Perry Williams, Cambridge: Cambridge University Press, 1992, 170–88.

Wernicke, Erich. 'Zur Geschichte des Diphtherieserums.' *Zeitschrift für ärztliche Fortbildung* 80, no. 5 (1931): 159–60.

Wittgenstein, Ludwig. *Tractatus Logico-Philosophicus.* Translated by Charles Ogden. London: Kegan Paul, Trench, Trubner & Co, 1922.

Worboys, Michael. *Spreading Germs: Disease Theories and Medical Practice in Britain, 1865–1900.* Cambridge: Cambridge University Press, 2000.

Zolot-Nisky. 'Revers de la médaille: ce que disent les adversaires de la sérothérapie.' *Lyon médical* 79 (1895).

Index

About the Author

Maître de conférences, **Jonathan Simon** teaches history and philosophy of science at the *Université de Lorraine* in Nancy, France. Trained in the field in England and the US, he holds a PhD in the history of chemistry from the University of Pittsburgh. He has published widely in the history and philosophy of chemistry and pharmacy, including *Chemistry, Pharmacy and Revolution in France, 1777–1809* in 2005 and *Chemistry: the impure science* with Bernadette Bensaude-Vincent in 2008. Jonathan Simon is a member of the Archives Poincaré in Nancy (UMR 7117) and is currently developing his research in the philosophy of technology related to pharmacy.

www.ingramcontent.com/pod-product-compliance
Ingram Content Group UK Ltd.
Pitfield, Milton Keynes, MK11 3LW, UK
UKHW020208290926
15470UKWH00001B/77

9 781498 531474